DRUG DERIVATIZA

HALF-LIFE

DR. R. K. AGRAWAL
Professor

Submitted By
VIVEK GUPTA
Enrolment No.:
SGVU092803653

Draft Contents

List of Figures	**I**
List of Tables	**VI**
List of Abbreviations	**VIII**
Abstract	**X**
Chapters	**Page No.**
1. Introduction	**01**
2. Drug Profile	**80**
3. Materials & Methods	**122**
4. *In-vitro* & *In-vivo* Studies	**172**
5. Summary & Conclusion	**212**
6. Recommendations	**225**
7. Publications	**226**

Acknowledgement

First of all, I sincerely want to thank my advisor Dr. R. K. Agrawal and Dr. A. K. Shrivastava for their guidance, support and encouragement. They gave me constructive criticisms as well as rewarding praises, which motivated and trained me to improve the quality of my research. They have also been a great role model and I undoubtedly intend to use what I have learned from them as I move forward in my career. I feel immense pleasure in expressing my sincere gratitude towards them.

This work is the wealth of experience and knowledge that is generated within the portals of Gyan Vihar School of Pharmacy, Suresh Gyan Vihar University, Jaipur which enlightened my path to complete my dissertation; otherwise, it would not have been possible.

I would like to convey my sincere thanks to Dr. S. C. Dewedi, Dean Research, S.G.V.U. and Dr. Ashish Sharma, Professor, Gyan Vihar School of Pharmacy for their erudite guidance, valuable suggestion & inspiration.

I mention my special thanks to Mr. Sunil Sharma, Honourable President, Suresh Gyan Vihar University, for providing facilities and infrastructure to carry out this work.

I submit my very sincere thanks to Dr. Sudhansu Sharma, Honourable Chief Mentor, Suresh Gyan Vihar University, for his continuous motivation.

I sincerely express my heartfelt thanks to all my colleagues and supporting staff of Gyan Vihar School of Pharmacy, without their blessing this work would have not been possible.

I am also thankful to my students Abhilasha Balani, Vinod Saini, Navratan Shrimal and Komal Sharma, they helped me in my dissertation work in numerous ways.

Finally, and most importantly, I would like to express much gratitude and love to my wife & son. Without their patience and love, I would not have been able to complete this work.

Above all my heartfelt veneration goes to my caring Mother and Almighty God, who are an integral part of my life, for their love, care, patience, inspiration, moral support and trust on me and well wishes they had bestowed upon me.

Last but not least, I would like to convey thanks to each of them who directly or indirectly help in completion of this work and whose name cannot be mentioned.

(Vivek Gupta)

List of Figures

Page No.

1.1 Fate of drug administered in body... .. 3

1.2 Mean serum IFN-α concentrations after a single 36×10^6 U dose as an intravenous infusion (O) or an intramuscular (X) or subcutaneous (Δ) injection...................... ..12

1.3 Relationship between frequency of dosing and maximum plasma concentrations 15

1.4 Testosterone hydroxyl group is protected by methyl group from Metabolism...............23

1.5 The use of a steric shield to protect the antirheumatic agent D 1927..........................25

1.6 Isosteric replacement of a methyl group with an amino group.................................25

1.7 Introducing a pyrrole ring as a bioisostere for an amide group................................27

1.8 Reduction of neighbouring group participation with an electron withdrawing group.......28

1.9 Stereoelectronic modifications which make lidocaine a longer lasting,local anaesthetic compared with procaine...29

1.10 Metabolic blocking by the addition of a methyl substituent.................................29

1.11 The use of fluorine substituents as metabolic blockers...30

1.12 Replacing metabolically labile groups...31

1.13 Salbutamol and noradrenaline...32

1.14 Metabolic methylation of a noradrenaline analogue……………………………………32

1.15 Increasing stability in antifungal agent……………………………………………. …..34

1.16 Stabilizing an aromatic or heteroaromatic methyl substituent by adding
a nitrogen to the ring……………………………………………………………………35

1.17 Ringsdorf model of synthetic polymer drugs……………………………………………..36

1.18 Biodegradable bonds used to conjugate bioactive molecules to polymer backbones…….37

1.19 Typical end-group polymer-drug conjugate based on PEG modifications………………40

1.20: The Dendritic Structure……………………………………………………………..45

1.21: Divergent Dendrimer Growth……………………………………………………… ...51

1.22: Correlation between intrinsic viscosity and Molecular weight………………………. 52

1.23: Dendrimer conformation……………………………………………………………54

1.24: Three-dimensional structure of a G6-PAMAM dendrimer, under different pH……........55

1.25: Two-dimensional depiction of conformational changes upon different pH of a carboxy terminated PPI-dendrimer…………………………………………………………...56

1.26: Proposed scheme for solvation of a dendrimer under different solvent conditions……..57

1.27: The three-dimensional conformational change of a PPI dendrimer upon increasing ionic strength……………………………………………………………………………58

1.28: Dendrimer at different concentrations…………………………………………………...59

1.29: Structures of biocompatible dendrimers that have been tested for drug delivery applications...61

1.30: The encapsulation of anticancer drugs methotraxate (left) and 5-fluorouracil (right) into PEGylated generation 3 and 4 PAMAM dendrimers..63

1.31: Dendrimer involved in gene transfection..68

2.1 Infrared absorption spectrum of sodium cloxacillin monohydrate..............................82

2.2 NMR spectrum of sodium cloxacillin monohydrate..83

2.3: FTIR Spectrum of Cloxacillin Sodium...92

2.4 Infrared Spectra of cephalexin monohydrate (potassium bromide disc)........................95

2.5 NMR spectrum of Cephalexin Monohydrate (D_2O + trifluoroacetic acid).....................96

2.6: FTIR Spectrum of Cephalexin...106

2.7 Infrared spectra of ciprofloxacin...108

2.8 H^1-NMR spectra of ciprofloxacin in D_2O..109

2.9: FTIR Spectrum of Ciprofloxacin...119

3.1: Schematic of divergent synthesis of dendrimers...122

3.2: Schematic of convergent synthesis of dendrimers..123

3.3. Structure of final derivatized cloxacillin..129

3.4 Structure of final derivatized cephalexin...130

3.5 Structure of final derivatized ciprofloxacin...131

4.1 Scanning electron micrograph of *S. aureus*...177

4.2 Calibration curve of cloxacillin in drug free control plasma...189

4.3 HPLC analysis of Plasma Blank for cloxacillin...189

4.4 HPLC analysis of Plasma with cloxacillin...190

4.5 HPLC analysis of Plasma with DDC...190

4.6 HPLC analysis of Plasma with DDC & Cloxacillin...191

4.7 Mean plasma concentrations of cloxacillin and derivatized cloxacillin following intravenous administration...193

4.8 Mean plasma concentrations of cloxacillin and derivatized cloxacillin following intravenous administration (log scale)...193

4.9 Calibration curve of cephalexin in drug free control plasma...196

4.10 HPLC analysis of Plasma Blank for cephalexin...196

4.11 HPLC analysis of Plasma with cephalexin...197

4.12 HPLC analysis of Plasma with DDC...197

4.13 Plasma with DDC & Cephalexin..198

4.14 Mean plasma concentrations of cephalexin and derivatized cephalexin following intravenous administration..200

4.15 Mean plasma concentrations of cephalexin and derivatized cephalexin following intravenous administration (log scale)..200

4.16 Calibration curve of ciprofloxacin in drug free control plasma..............................203

4.17 HPLC analysis of Plasma Blank for Ciprofloxacin..203

4.18 HPLC analysis of Plasma with ciprofloxacin...204

4.19 HPLC analysis of Plasma with DDC..204

4.20 HPLC analysis of Plasma with DDC & Ciprofloxacin......................................205

4.21 Mean plasma concentrations of ciprofloxacin and derivatized ciprofloxacin following intravenous administration..207

4.22 Mean plasma concentrations of ciprofloxacin and derivatized ciprofloxacin following intravenous administration (log scale)..207

List of Tables

Page No.

1.1 Percentage of Dose Lost as a Function of Number of Half-Lives..........................14

1.2 Properties of Dendrimer and linear polymers.. ...53

3.1 Solubility data of Intermediates and derivatized drugs...................................136

3.2 Physicochemical data of synthesized compounds... 137

3.3 Interpretation of FTIR spectra of E.D.T.A. (G 0)..138

3.4 Interpretation of FTIR spectra of E.D.T.A. (G 1.0)..140

3.5 Interpretation of FTIR spectra of E.D.T.A. (G 1.5)..141

3.6 Interpretation of H^1-NMR of G1.5 compound..142

3.7 Interpretation of FTIR of compound G 2.0..144

3.8 Interpretation of FTIR spectra of compound G 2.5..145

3.9 Interpretation of H^1-NMR spectra of compound G 2.5................................ 146

3.10 Interpretation of FTIR of compound G 3.0..148

3.11 Interpretation of H^1-NMR spectra of compound G 3.0.................................149

3.12 Interpretation of FTIR of Cloxacillin conjugated PEG 4000............................150

3.13 Interpretation of H^1-NMR of Cloxacillin conjugated PEG 4000........................151

3.14 Interpretation of FTIR of Cloxacillin-conjugated PEG-dendrimer.......................153

3.15 Interpretation of H^1-NMR of Cloxacillin-conjugated PEG-dendrimer............... 154

3.16 Interpretation of FTIR of Cephalexin conjugated PEG 4000............................155

3.17 Interpretation of H^1-NMR of Cephalexin conjugated PEG 4000.................... 156

3.18 Interpretation of FTIR of Cephalexin-conjugated PEG-dendrimer.....................158

3.19 Interpretation of H^1-NMR of Cephalexin-conjugated PEG-dendrimer.................159

3.20 Interpretation of FTIR of Ciprofloxacin conjugated PEG 4000.........................160

3.21 Interpretation of H^1-NMR of Ciprofloxacin conjugated PEG 4000....................161

3.22 Interpretation of FTIR of Ciprofloxacin-conjugated PEG-dendrimer...................163

3.23 Interpretation of H^1-NMR of Ciprofloxacin-conjugated PEG-dendrimer..............164

4.1 Comparative antibacterial study of cloxacillin and derivatized cloxacillin................184
4.2 Comparative antibacterial study of cephalexin and derivatized cephalexin...............184
4.3 Comparative antibacterial study of ciprofloxacin and derivatized ciprofloxacin.........185
4.4 Cloxacillin Concentration in drug free control plasma Vs Mean Area.....................188
4.5 Concentrations of cloxacillin and cloxacillin released from DDC obtained by HPLC analysis of plasma samples collected at different time intervals................192
4.6 Cephalexin concentrations in drug free control plasma Vs. Mean Area....................195
4.7 Concentrations of cephalexin and cephalexin released from DDC obtained by HPLC analysis of plasma samples collected at different time intervals...............199
4.8 Ciprofloxacin concentrations in drug free control plasma vs. Mean Area..................202
4.9 Concentrations of ciprofloxacin and ciprofloxacin released from DDC obtained by HPLC analysis of plasma samples collected at different time intervals............ ...206
4.10 Half-life Enhancement Data from In-vivo Experiments...................................209
5.1 Increase in molecular weight after drug derivatization.......................................221

List of Abbreviations

$t_{1/2}$	Half-life
CL	Clearance
F	Bioavailability
AUC	Area Under Curve
ER	Extraction Ratio
CYP	Cytochrome P450
V	Volume of Distribution
AUMC	Area Under Moment Curve
MEC	Minimum effective concentration
MTC	Minimum toxic concentration
C_{SS}	Steady-state concentrations
MRTC	Mean residence time in the central compartment
MRT	Mean residence time in the body
e.w.g.	electron withdrawing group
DDS	Drug Delivery Systems
PEG	Polyethyleneglycol
PAMAM	Poly (amidoamine) dendrimers
PAMAMOS	Poly (amidoamine-organosilicon) dendrimers
PPI	Poly (Propylene Imine) dendrimers
POPAM	Poly (Propylene Amine) dendrimers
THF	Tetrahydrofuran

PDT	Photodynamic Therapy
FTIR	Fourier Transform Infrared Spectroscopy
H^1-NMR	Proton Nuclear Magnetic Resonance
HPLC	High Performance Liquid Chromatography
RSD	Relative standard deviation
EDTA	Ethylenediaminetetraaceticacid
DCC	Dicyclohexyl carbidoimide
DCU	Dicyclohexylurea
G	Dendrimer Generation
NPC	Pera-nitrophenylchloroformate
DMAP	4-dimethylaminopyridine
MHA	Mueller Hinton Agar
MHB	Mueller Hinton Broth
DDC	Drug Dendrimer Complex

ABSTRACT

Some of the drugs are having very short half-life, to compensate this problem it is common practice to increase the dosage, frequency or prolongation of administration of drug to maintain effective therapeutic concentration in patient. In this study a drug delivery scaffold was designed and synthesized based on polyethylene glycol (PEG)-ethylene diamine tetra acetic acid (EDTA) based poly(amidoamine) (PAMAM) star polymer (with 16 primary amine group on surface). Cloxacillin, Cephalexin and Ciprofloxacin were used as a model drugs having short half life to conjugate with PEGylated dendrimer. These drugs were coupled to star polymer via ester bond. Fourier transform infrared spectroscopy (FT-IR) and proton nuclear magnetic resonance (^{1}H-NMR) was used to characterize the intermediate and drug-star-polymer conjugates. In-vitro activity of derivatized drugs compared to standard drug alone, it was found that zone of inhibition obtained by both category of drugs (standard and derivatized drugs) are almost similar. That means drug derivatization does not altering the antibacterial activity of drugs. To investigate pharmacokinetic parameters, selected drugs alone and modified drugs [(Drug-PEG)$_{16}$-Dendrimer] were intravenously injected into rats. All the modified drugs demonstrated a dramatic increase in half-life than drugs alone. These studies suggest the use of these new PEG based EDTA core dendrimer support as a valuable alternative for enhancing biological half-life of drugs.

The duration of action of a drug is known as its half life ($t_{1/2}$). This is the period of time required for the concentration or amount of drug in the body to be reduced by one-half. We usually consider the half life of a drug in relation to the amount of the drug in plasma. A drug's plasma half-life depends on how quickly the drug is eliminated from the plasma. A drug molecule that leaves plasma may have any of several fates. It can be eliminated from the body or it can be translocated to another body fluid compartment such as the intracellular fluid or it can be destroyed in the blood. The removal of a drug from the plasma is known as clearance and the distribution of the drug in various body tissues is known as the volume of distribution. Both of these pharmacokinetic parameters are important in determining the half life of a drug.

Experimentally the half life can be determined by giving a single dose, usually intravenously and then the concentration of the drug in the plasma is measured at regular intervals. The concentration of the drug will reach a peak value in the plasma and will then fall as the drug clearance progresses.

The time taken for the plasma concentration to halve is the half life of that drug. Some drugs like ibuprofen have very short half lives, others like warfarin and digoxin, take much longer time to eliminate from the plasma resulting in a long half life. So drugs like ibuprofen that are cleared from the blood more rapidly than others need to be given in regular doses to build up and maintain a high enough concentration in the blood to be therapeutically effective.

As repeated doses of a drug are administered its plasma concentration builds up and reaches what is known as a steady state. This is when the amount of drug in the plasma has built up to a concentration level that is therapeutically effective and as long as regular doses are administered to balance the amount of drug being cleared the drug will continue to be active. The time taken to reach the steady state is about five times the half life of a drug. Drugs like digoxin and warfarin with a long half life will take longer to reach a steady state than drugs with a shorter half life.

Sometimes a loading dose may be administered so that a steady state is reached more quickly than smaller 'maintenance' doses are given to ensure that the drug levels stay within the steady state.

1.1 PHARMACOKINETIC PARAMETERS AFFECTING DRUG'S HALF-LIFE

Absorption, distribution, and elimination processes begin when a dose is administered and may govern the appearance of any therapeutic effect (Fig.1.1). Pharmacokinetics is used to quantitate these processes. Apart from its usefulness in explaining the safety and toxicity assessment data, pharmacokinetic analysis is used primarily to design appropriate dosing regimens and also to quantitatively define drug disposition. The term pharmacokinetics can be defined as what the body does to the drug. The parallel term, pharmacodynamics, can be defined as what the drug does to the body. A fundamental hypothesis of pharmacokinetics is that a relationship exists between a pharmacologic or toxic effect of a drug and the concentration of the drug in a readily accessible site of the body (e.g., blood). This hypothesis has been documented for many drugs[1, 2]; although for some drugs no clear relationship has been found between pharmacologic effect and plasma or blood concentrations.

Among many pharmacokinetic parameters, that can be determined when defining pharmacokinetics of a new drug substance are clearance, effective concentration range, extent of availability, fraction of the available dose excreted unchanged, concentration ratio, toxic concentration, extent of protein binding, volume of distribution and rate of availability.

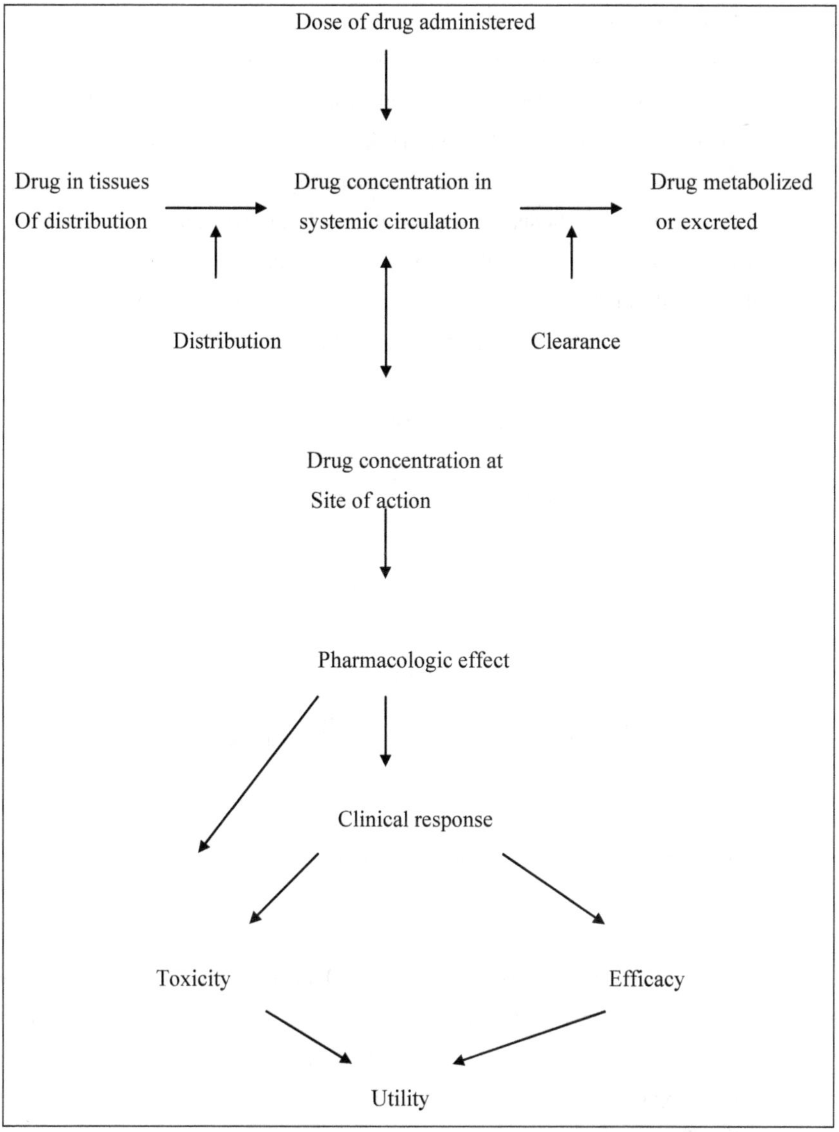

Figure 1.1 Fate of drug administered in body

1.1.1 Clearance

Clearance (CL) is the measure of the ability of the body to eliminate a drug. Initially, clearance will be looked at from a physiological point of view. The rate of presentation of a drug to a drug elimination organ is the product of organ blood flow (Q) and the concentration of drug in the arterial blood entering the organ (C_A). The rate of exit of a drug from the drug-elimination organ is the product of the organ blood flow (Q) and the concentration of the drug in the venous blood leaving the organ (Cv). By mass balance, the rate of elimination (or extraction) of a drug by a drug-elimination organ is the difference between the rate of presentation and the rate of exit.

$$\text{Rate of presentation} = QC_A \text{..................} 1$$

$$\text{Rate of exit} = QC_V \text{..........................} 2$$

$$\text{Rate of elimination} = QCA - QC_V$$

$$= Q\,(C_A - C_V) \text{..............} 3$$

The extraction ratio (ER) of an organ can be defined as the ratio of the rate of elimination to the rate of presentation.

Extraction ratio = rate of elimination/ rate of presentation

$$ER = Q\,(C_A - C_V) / QC_A \text{..} 4$$

The maximum possible extraction ratio is 1.0 when no drug emerges into the venous blood upon presentation to the eliminating organ (i.e., $C_V = 0$). The lowest possible extraction ratio is zero, when the entire drug passing through the potential drug-eliminating organ appears in the venous blood (i.e., $C_V = C_A$). Drugs with an extraction ratio of more than 0.7 are by convention considered as high extraction ratio drugs, whereas those with an extraction ratio of less than 0.3 are considered as low extraction ratio drugs.

The product of organ blood flow and extraction ratio of an organ represents a rate at which a certain volume of blood is completely cleared of a drug. This expression defines the organ clearance (CL_{organ}) of a drug.

$$CL_{organ} = QER = Q\,(C_A\text{-}C_V)/\,C_A \text{ ....5}$$

From equation 3 and 5, one can see that clearance is proportionality constant between rate of elimination and the arterial drug concentration.

At steady state, by definition, rate in equal's rate out. Rate is given by the dosing rate (Dose/τ, i.e., dose divided by dosing interval τ) multiplied by the drug availability F, whereas rate out is the rate of elimination (clearance multiplied by the systemic concentration C).

$$\text{Rate in} = \text{Rate out..................6}$$

$$F\,(\text{Dose}/\,\tau) = CL\,(C)\text{.....................7}$$

When equation 7 is integrated over time from zero to infinity, equation 8 results.

$$F\,(\text{Dose}) = CL\,(AUC)\text{.................8}$$

Where AUC is the area under the concentration time curve and F is the fraction of dose available to the systemic circulation.

Clearance may be calculated as the available dose divided by the area under the systemic drug concentration curve.

$$CL = F\,(\text{Dose})/\,AUC\text{.................9}$$

The maximum value for organ clearance is limited by the blood flow to the organ (i.e., extraction ratio is 1). The average blood flow to the kidneys is approximately 66 L/h and to the liver, approximately 81 L/h Clearance can occur in many sites in the body and is generally additive. Elimination of a drug may occur as a result of processes occurring in the liver, the kidney, and other organs. The total systemic clearance will be the sum of the individual organ clearances.

$$CL_{total} = CL_{hepatic} + CL_{renal} + CL_{other} \ldots\ldots\ldots\ldots 10$$

Among the many organs that are capable of eliminating drugs, the liver, in general, has the highest metabolic capability. Drug molecules in blood are bound to blood cells and plasma proteins such as albumin and alpha-acid glycoprotein. Yet only unbound drug molecules can pass through hepatic membranes into hepatocytes, where they are metabolized by hepatic enzymes or transported into the bile. Thus to be eliminated, drug molecules must partition out of the red blood cells and dissociate from plasma proteins to become unbound or free drug molecules. Because unbound drug molecules are free to partition into and out of the blood cells and hepatocytes, there is equilibrium of free drug concentration between the blood cells, the plasma, and the hepatocytes. The ratio between unbound drug concentration and the total drug concentration constitutes the fraction unbound (f_u)

Fraction unbound = unbound drug concentration / total drug concentration

Or

$$F_u = C_u / C \ldots\ldots\ldots\ldots\ldots\ldots 11$$

Because an equilibrium exists between the unbound drug molecules in the blood cells and the plasma, the rate of elimination of unbound drugs is the same in the whole blood as in the plasma at steady state. Thus,

$$CL_pC_p = CL_bC_b = CL_uC_u \ldots\ldots\ldots\ldots\ldots\ldots 12$$

Where the subscripts p, b, and u refer to plasma, blood, and unbound, respectively. From the material presented so far, one may intuitively imagine that hepatic drug clearance will be influenced by hepatic blood flow, fraction unbound, and intrinsic clearance; that is, the intrinsic ability of the organ to clear unbound drug. The simplest model that describes hepatic clearance in terms of these physiological parameters is the well stirred model [3]. Assuming instantaneous and complete mixing, the well-stirred model states that hepatic clearance (with respect to blood concentration) is

$$CL_{hep} = Q_{hep}f_uCL / Q_{hep} + (f_uCL_{int}) \ldots\ldots 13$$

f_u is calculated from unbound and total concentration in whole blood. Equation 5 advises that hepatic clearance is the product of hepatic blood flow and hepatic extraction ratio. Therefore, as shown in Equation 13, the hepatic extraction ratio is

$$ER_{hep} = f_uCL_{int} / Q_{hep} + (f_uCL_{int}) \ldots\ldots 14$$

By examining Equations 13 and 14, one finds that for drugs with a high extraction ratio *(i.e.,* ER approaches 1.0), f_uCL_{int} is much greater than Q_{hep} and clearance approaches Q_{hep} In other words, the clearance for a high extraction ratio drug, imipramine for example, is perfusion rate limited. For drugs with a low extraction ratio (i.e., ER approaches zero), Q_{hep} is much greater than f_uCL_{int} and clearance is approximated by $f_uCL_{int.}$ An example of a low extraction ratio drug is acetaminophen.

The intrinsic ability of an organ to clear a drug is directly proportional to the activity of the metabolic enzymes in the organ. Such metabolic processes, both in vitro and in vivo, are characterized by Michaelis-Menten kinetics:

$$\text{Rate of metabolism} = V_{MAX}C / (K_M + C) \ldots\ldots 15$$

In which $V_{MAX,}$ the maximum rate at which metabolism can proceed, is proportional to the total concentration of enzyme. K_M is the Michaelis-Menten constant corresponding to the drug concentration that yields one-half of the maximum rate of metabolism. Dividing both sides of Equation15 by the systemic concentration C yields

Rate of metabolism/C = $CL_{metabolism} = V_{MAX}C / (K_M + C)$………………..16

Because identification of a saturable process occurs only for low extraction ratio compounds (i.e., $CL_{metabolism} = f_u\, CL_{int}$), the relationship between classical enzyme and pharmacokinetics is revealed:

$f_u\, CL_{int} = V_{MAX} / (K_M + C)$……………………………..17

Because V_{MAX} and K_M can be obtained from in vitro metabolism experiments, development scientists may reasonably predict the in vivo clearance parameter of a low or intermediate extraction ratio drug from in vitro data, by use of Equations13 and17. By use of appropriate scaling factors, the in vivo clearance parameter in humans can be approximated from in vitro metabolism data from other species[4, 5].

The kidneys are also important drug eliminating organs. Renal clearance ($CL\tau$) is a proportionality term between urinary excretion rate and systemic concentration. By integrating Equation 18a over time from zero to infinity, one obtains renal clearance, which is the ratio of the total amount of the drug excreted unchanged to the area under the systemic concentration curve. The total amount of drug excreted unchanged can be measured experimentally or can be calculated from the dose, if the fraction of the available dose excreted unchanged (fe) is known.

$CL\tau$ = Urinary excretion rate/C……………………………………………18a

= Total amount of drug excreted unchanged/AUC…………………18b

= f_e [F (Dose)]/AUC…………………………………………………18c

It is obvious from the preceding arguments that the conceptual approach to clearance requires measurements of blood concentrations. Yet, bioanalytical measurements are often carried out in plasma because of the ease of sample handling. However, measuring the blood to plasma ratio allows one to convert clearance values, determined in plasma, to their corresponding blood values by use of Equation 12.

1.1.2 Bioavailability

The bioavailability of a drug product through various routes of administration is defined as the fraction of unchanged drug that is absorbed intact and then reaches the site of action; or the systemic circulation following administration by any route. For an intravenous dose of a drug, bioavailability is defined as unity. For drugs administered by other routes of administration, bioavailability is often less than unity. Incomplete bioavailability may be attributed to a number of factors that can be subdivided into categories of dosage-form effects, membrane effects, and site of administration effects. Obviously, the route of administration that offers maximum bioavailability is the direct input at the site of action for which the drug is developed. This arrangement may be difficult to achieve because the site of action is not known for disease states and, in other cases, the site of action may be completely inaccessible, even when the drug is placed into the blood stream. The most commonly used route is oral administration. However, orally administered drugs may decompose in the fluids of the gastrointestinal lumen, or be metabolized as they pass through the gastrointestinal membrane. In addition, once a drug passes into the hepatic portal vein, it may be cleared by the liver before entering into the general circulation. The loss of drug as it passes through drug-eliminating organs for the time is known as the ***first-pass effect.***

The fraction of an oral dose available to the systemic circulation, considering both absorption and the first-pass effect, can be found by comparing the ratio of AUCs after oral and intravenous dosing.

$$F = AUC_{oral} / AUC_{i.v..} \quad \text{.............................19}$$

If an assumption is made that all of a drug dose is absorbed through the gastrointestinal tract intact, and that the only extraction takes place at the liver, then the maximum bioavailability F_{max} is

$$F_{max} = 1 - ER_{hep} \quad \text{.........20}$$

From Equations 5 and 20, one can derive the following relationship for F_{max}

$$F_{max} = 1 - (CL_{hep} / Q_{hep}) \quad \text{.........21}$$

For high extraction ratio drugs, where CL_{hep} approaches Q_{hep}, F_{max} will be small. For low extraction ratio drugs, Q_{hep} is much greater than CL_{hep} and F_{max} will approximate one. Recently bioavailability and clearance data obtained from a crossover study of cyclosporine kinetics before and after rifampin dosing revealed a new understanding of drug metabolism and disposition of the compound[6]. Healthy volunteers were given cyclosporine, intravenously and orally, before and after CYP3A (P450 3A) enzymes were introduced by rifampin. As expected, the blood clearance of cyclosporine increased from 0.31 to 0.42 L h^{-1} Kg^{-1} as a result of the induction of the drug's metabolizing enzymes (i.e., an increase in V_{max} in Equation 15). There was no change in volume of distribution, but there was a dramatic decrease in bioavailability from 27% to 10% in these individuals.

A decrease in bioavailability is to be expected because cyclosporine undergoes some first-pass metabolism as it goes through the liver after oral dosing. However, if one predicts on the basis of pharmacokinetics what the maximum bioavailability [as calculated by Equation 21 would be before and after rifampin dosing, the maximum bioavailability would decrease from 77% to 68%. Thus, there would be an expected cyclosporine bioavilability decrease of approximately 12% just on the basis of clearance changes resulting from inducing CYP3A enzymes in the liver. In fact, there was a bioavailability decrease of 60%. Furthermore, bioavailability was significantly less than would be predicted at maximum. Although some of that lower bioavailability was attributed to formulation effects, the discrepancy between the theoretical maximum availability and the achievable bioavailability of cyclosporine remained a question.

However, on the basis of new findings during the last several years about the high prevalence of CYP3A isozymes in the gut, significant metabolism of cyclosporine in the gut as well as in the liver was speculated. This hypothesis can consistently explain the significantly lower bioavailability that would be predicted, even if all of the drug could be absorbed into the blood stream. This finding, particularly quantification of the magnitude of gut metabolism (more than two-thirds of the total metabolism for an oral dose of cyclosporine occurs in the gut), would not have been realized, had pharmacokinetics not been used in the analysis of the given data.

1.1.3 Volume of Distribution

The volume of distribution (V) relates the amount of drug in the body to the concentration of drug in the blood or plasma, depending on the fluid measured. At its simplest, this relationship is defined by Equation 22:

$$V = \text{amount of drug in body}/C \quad \ldots\ldots 22$$

At equilibrium, the distribution of a drug within the body depends on binding to blood cells, plasma proteins, and tissue components. Only the unbound drug is capable of entering and leaving the plasma and tissue compartments. A memory aid for this relationship can be summarized by the expression

$$V = V_P + V_{TW}\, f_u / f_{u\,T} \quad \ldots\ldots 23$$

Where V_P is the volume of plasma, V_{TW} is the aqueous volume outside plasma, f_u is the fraction unbound in plasma, and $f_{u\,T}$ is the fraction unbound in tissue. Thus, a drug that has a high degree of binding to plasma proteins (i.e., low f_u) will generally exhibit a small of distribution. Unlike plasma protein binding, tissue binding of a drug cannot be measured directly. Generally, this parameter is assumed to be constant unless indicated otherwise.

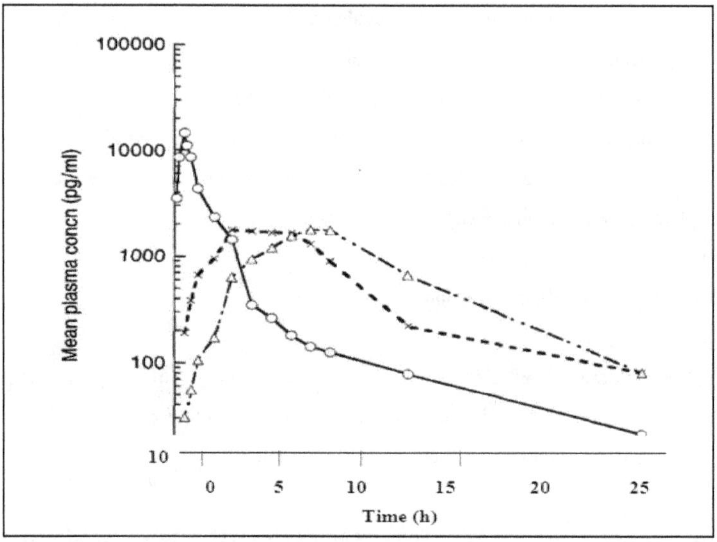

Figure 1.2 Mean serum IFN-α concentrations after a single 36 × 10^6 U dose as an intravenous infusion (O) or an intramuscular (X) or subcutaneous (Δ) injection[7].

In Equation 22, the body is considered as a single homogeneous pool of body fluids as described above for digoxin. For most drugs, however, two or three distinct pools of distribution space appear to exist. This condition results in a time-dependent decrease in the measurable blood or plasma concentration, which reflects distribution into other body pools independent of the body's ability to eliminate the drug. Figure 1.2 describes mean serum IFN-α concentrations after a 40-min intravenous infusion as well as after intra-muscular and subcutaneous injections of the same dose. Note the logarithmic biphasic nature of the mean plasma concentration-time curve after the intravenous infusion. This biphasic nature represents both the distribution and elimination processes.

Generally, comparisons of volume of distribution are made by use of a parameter designated as the volume of distribution at steady state (Vss), which reflects the sum of the volumes of all the pools into which a drug may distribute. Vss can be calculated from the area under the moment curve (AUMC) and the area under the curve (AUC) as defined by Benet and Galeazzi[8]:

$$V_{SS} = Dose_{i.v.} AUMC/AUC^2 \qquad \text{......24}$$

AUMC can be calculated from areas under a plot of concentration vs. time. Both AUC and AUMC may be calculated from the coefficients and exponents of the equations used to describe the multicompartment nature of drug kinetics as depicted in Fig.1.2.

In addition to the three parameters, clearance (CL), bioavailability(F) and volume of distribution (V) discussed previously, a fourth parameter, **half-life ($t_{1/2}$)**, is also crucial in therapeutics. Clearance defines the dosing rate, bioavailability defines dose adjustment, and half-life defines the dosing interval. Volume of distribution defines the loading dose.

1.1.4 Dosing Rate

As discussed in Equation 6, rate of presentation equals rate of exit at steady rate. Whereas rate of presentation is the product of bioavailability and dosing rate, rate of exit is the product of clearance and average (steady-state) concentration. By replacing the average concentration with the target concentration, the dosing rate can be computed with known values of bioavailability and clearance.

$$\text{Rate in} = \text{rate out} \qquad \text{......6}$$

$$\text{Bioavailability} \times \text{dosing rate} = \text{Clearance} \times \text{average concentration} \qquad \text{......7a}$$

$$F\,(\text{dosing rate}) = CL\,(C_{target}) \qquad \text{......7b}$$

1.1.5 Dose Adjustment

There is often a therapeutic concentration range of drug in the blood that is necessary to elicit a clinical effect without causing drug toxicity. The boundaries of this range are set by the minimum effective concentration (MEC) and the minimum toxic concentration (MTC). For example, to maintain a steady rate of presentation of 100 mg/min, one can administer either a completely bioavailable intravenous (i.v.) infusion at 100 mg/min or a sustained release oral dosage form with 50% bioavailability at 200mg/min. As shown in Equations 7a and 7b, the actual dosing rate depends on the bioavailability of the dosage form. For proper dosing adjustment, the bioavailability (F) of a given dosage form stands as a must-know parameter in therapeutics.

1.1.6 Dosing Interval

Half-life ($t_{1/2}$) is an extremely useful kinetic parameter in terms of therapeutics, given that this parameter, together with therapeutic index, helps define the dosing interval at which drugs should be administered. By definition, half-life is the time required for 50% of the drug remaining in the body to be eliminated. In three and one-third half-lives, 90% of the dose would have been eliminated. Table 2 shows the percentage of dose lost in different numbers of half-lives.

Table 1.1 Percentage of Dose Lost as a Function of Number of Half-Lives

Number of Half-Lives	Dose Lost (%)
1	50
2	75
3	87.5
3.3	90
4	93.8
5	96.9

If the dosing interval is long relative to the half-life, large fluctuations in drug concentration will occur. On the other hand, if the dosing interval is short relative to half-life, significant accumulation will occur. The half-life parameter also allows one to predict drug accumulation within the body and quantifies the approach to plateau that occurs with multiple dosing and constant rates of infusion. Conventionally, three and one third half-lives are used as the time required achieving steady state under constant infusion. The concentration level achieved after this time is already 90%of the steady-state concentration and, clinically, it is difficult to distinguish a 10% difference in concentrations.

After determining the extent of oral drug bioavailability, half-life is probably the next most important parameter in terms of deciding the appropriateness of a drug for further development. Drugs with very short half-lives create problems in maintaining steady-state concentrations in the therapeutic range. Thus, a successful drug product with a short half-life will require a dosage form that allows a relatively constant prolonged input. Drugs with a very long half-life are favored in terms of efficacy considerations; however, this long half-life may be a negative characteristic in terms of toxicity considerations. Figure 1.3 illustrates the importance of half-life in defining the dosing interval

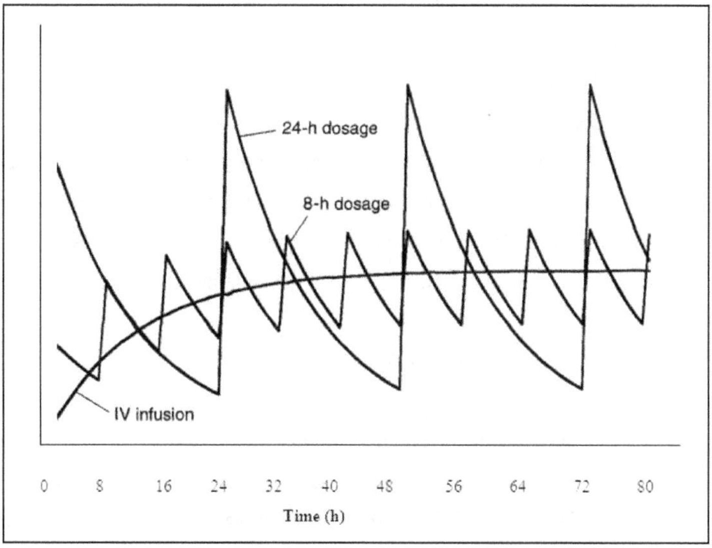

Figure1.3 Relationship between frequency of dosing and maximum plasma concentrations when a steady-state plasma level of 15 μg/mL is desired. The time course of plasma concentrations for 43.2 mg/h intravenous infusion, and 8-hourly 340 mg oral dose, and a 24-hourly 1020 mg oral dose are depicted.

Figure 1.3 depicts the relationship between the frequency of theophylline dosing and the plasma concentration time course when a steady-state theophylline plasma level of 15 μg/mL is desired. The smoothly rising curve shows the plasma concentration achieved with an i.v. infusion of 43.2 mg/h to a patient exhibiting an average theophylline clearance of 0.69 mL/min.kg. The steady state theophylline plasma level achieved is midway within the therapeutic concentration range of 10-20 μg/mL. The figure also depicts the time courses for 8-hourly administration of 340 mg and 24 hourly administration of 1020 mg, assuming that these dose are administered in an immediate release dosage form. In each case the mean steady state concentration is 15 μg/mL. However the peak to trough ratio and the concentrations achieved with once daily dosing (i.e., 1020 mg) of a rapidly released formulation would result in concentrations in the toxic range, exceeding 20 μg/mL for certain periods of time as well as concentration less than 10 μg/mL, for significant periods during each dosing interval. In contrast the 8 hourly dosing, which is approximately equivalent to the half-life of theophylline, shows a twofold range in peak to trough, and theophylline levels stay within the therapeutic plasma concentration range.

Although half-life is a very important parameter in therapeutics for defining the dosing interval, half-life can be a very misleading parameter when one is attempting to use pharmacokinetics as a tool in defining drug disposition. As depicted in Equation 25, half-life varies as a function of the two physiologically related parameters, volume and clearance.

$$t_{1/2} = 0.693\ (V/CL) \qquad \ldots 25$$

As clearance decreases, because of a disease process, half-life would be expected to increase. However, this reciprocal relationship is exact only when the disease does not change the volume of distribution. For example, as Klotz and coworkers have shown, the increase in half-life of diazepam with age does not result from a decrease in clearance but rather results from an increase in volume as the patient ages[9].

Clearance, a measure of the body's ability to eliminate the drug, does not significantly decrease with age for diazepam. However, when volume increases, fewer drugs is in the blood flowing to the liver and elimination can occur only for those molecules that come into contact with the liver. Thus the time that the drug remains in the body is increased. The half-life of Tolbutamide decreases in patients with acute viral hepatitis; that is; the drug appears to be eliminated faster by a diseased liver, the exact opposite from what one might expect. Here, the disease appears to decrease protein binding in both plasma and tissues, causing no change in volume of distribution but an increase in free fraction in the plasma, which results in an increase in total clearance and, subsequently, a decrease in half-life[10].

Equation 25 describes the half-life relationship for a drug that appears to follow single compartment body kinetics; that is, when the body is considered to be a single homogeneous pool of body fluids. However, many drugs appear to exhibit multiple distribution pools and therefore may have multiple half-lives (as was depicted in Fig.1.2 for IFN-a). Drugs with multiple half-lives are usually reported in the literature as having "distribution" and "terminal elimination" half-lives. Defining the "relevant" half-life in such situations has been addressed by Benet and coworkers[11, 12].

Consider the situation in which a drug is best described by a two-pool model, as has been suggested for IFN-a by Wills et al.[7]. The data in the Wills study were recalculated to represent the equation describing the concentration (ng/mL) of the drug after a 228 μg dose of IFN-a as a function of time (h), as given in equation 26.

$$C = 14.13e^{-1.04t} + 0.545e^{-0.136t} \qquad (26)$$

The disposition constants in the exponents of Equation 26 correspond to half-lives of 0.667 h (40 min) and 5.1 h. In the interferon literature, the 5.1-h half-life is generally referred to as the mean elimination half-life, whereas the 40-min half-life, if mentioned at all, is generally referred to as a distribution half-life. These representations may not be accurate; the relevance of a particular half-life may be defined in terms of the fraction of the clearance that is related to each half-life. Note in Equation 8 that clearance is inversely related to area under the drug concentration time curve (AUC).When the equation describing the time course of drug concentrations requires more than one exponential term, this circumstance can be represented by Equation 27. For an n-compartment pharmacokinetic model,

$$C = L_1 e^{-\lambda_1 t} + L_2 e^{-\lambda 2t} + \ldots\ldots + L_n e^{-\lambda nt} \ldots\ldots 27$$

AUC can be calculated as the ratio of coefficients and exponents as in Equation 28.

$$AUC = L_1/\lambda_1 + L_2/\lambda_2 + \ldots\ldots + L_n/\lambda_n \ldots\ldots 28$$

Calculating AUC for IFN-a as described in equation 26 yields

$$AUC\ (ngh^{-1}mL^{-1}) = \underset{(77\%)}{13.59} + \underset{(23\%)}{4.01}$$

Note that 77% of the AUC relates to the coefficient and exponent for the 40-min half-life, which suggests that the 5.1-h half-life is in fact a minor contributor to the prediction of steady-state concentrations of IFN-a. The importance of these fractional areas can be observed if Equation 7 is rearranged to predict steady-state concentrations (C_{SS}):

$$C_{SS} = F\ (Dose)/\ (\tau CL) \ldots\ldots 7c$$

Now, given that CL can be defined as given in Equation 9 as the relationship between an available single dose and AUC, Equation 7c becomes

$$C_{SS} = [F\ (Dose)]\ AUC/\tau\ [F\ (Dose)] \ldots\ldots 29$$

Thus, the ability to correctly predict C_{SS} is dependent on the accuracy of the measurement of AUC. If the 5.1-h half-life for IFN-a is ignored, the data of Wills et al. suggest that the value for AUC, and therefore the steady state concentration, will be underestimated by only 23%, given that this longer half-life represents a relatively small fraction of the total IFN-a clearance[7]. This error in drug concentrations could probably be ignored with confidence because a 23%difference may often be within analytical error for protein drugs, as well as within the day-to-day variability in a particular patient.

The above calculations assume that drug concentrations are important in defining the efficacy or toxicity of IFN-a. If this is true, the clinician can safely ignore the 5.1-h half-life in patients with normal elimination characteristics because little change in steady-state drug levels will be observed. However, it may be that the response, particularly toxicity, is related to the amount of drug in the body, rather than the systemic concentration. The amount in the body at steady state (Ass) is the product of the systemic concentration and the steady state volume of distribution:

$$Ass = Css\ Vss$$

As can be seen from Equation 24, the accurate calculation of Vss requires an understanding of how AUMC is related to the fractional area of each half-life. The complications of this relationship will not be discussed in this introductory chapter but the correct estimation of Vss is always significantly determined by the terminal half-life. More recently, Benet called multiple dosing half-lives, the half-life for a drug that is equivalent to the dosing interval to choose so that plasma concentrations (Equation 31) or amounts of drug in the body (Equation 32) will show a 50% drop during a dosing interval at a steady stat These parameters are defined in terms of the mean residence time in the central compartment (MRTC) and the mean residence time in the body (MRT).

$$t_{1/2MD}^{plasma} = 0.693\ MRTC \qquad \ldots\ldots 31$$

$$t_{1/2MD}^{amount} = 0.693\ MRTC \qquad \ldots\ldots 32$$

MRTC in a one-compartment body model is the inverse of the rate constant for elimination. In a multiple-compartment model, where the multiple dosing plasma half-life is useful, MTRC is given by the volume of the central compartment where drug concentrations are measured divided by clearance. MRT in Equation 32 is the ratio of AUMC/AUC.

1.1.7 Loading Dose

For drugs with long half-lives, the time to reach steady state is substantial. In these instances, it may be desirable to administer a loading dose that promptly raises the concentration of a drug in plasma to the projected steady-state value. In theory, only the amount of the loading dose needs to be computed, not the rate of its administration. To a first approximation, this is true. The amount of drug required to achieve a given steady state concentration in the plasma is the amount of drug that must be in the body when the desired steady state is reached. For intermittent dosage schemes, the amount is that at the average concentration. The volume of distribution is the proportionality factor that relates the total amount of drug in the body to the concentration in the plasma. If a loading dose is administered to achieve the desired steady-state concentration, then

$$\text{Loading dose} = \text{amount in the body at steady state} = C_{P,\,SS}\,V_{SS} \qquad \text{.......................33}$$

For most drugs, the loading dose can be given as a single dose by the chosen route of administration. However, for drugs that follow complicated a multicompartment model, the distribution phase cannot be ignored in the calculation of the loading dose. If the rate of absorption is rapid relative to distribution (this circumstance is always true for i.v. bolus administration), the concentration of drug in plasma that results from an appropriate loading dose can initially be considerably higher than desired. Severe toxicity may occur, albeit transiently. This may be particularly important, for example, in the administration of anti arrhythmic drugs, where an almost immediate toxic response is obtained when plasma concentrations exceed a particular level. Thus, although estimation of the amount of the loading dose may be quite correct, the rate of administration can be crucial in preventing excessive drug concentrations, and slow administration of an i.v. drug (over minutes rather than seconds) is almost always wise.

1.2 STRATEGIES TO MANAGE DRUG METABOLISM FOR ENHANCING HALF-LIFE

A variety of methods have been used to circumvent the rapid metabolism of certain drugs. These methods seek to improve drug therapy decreasing the overall extent of metabolism and increasing the duration of action. In some instances, these methods have provided increased site specificity.

1.2.1. Pharmaceutical strategies involve the use of different dosage forms to either avoid or compensate for rapid metabolism[13].

Sublingual tablets are useful for delivering drugs directly into the systemic circulation and bypassing hepatic first-pass metabolism. **Nitroglycerin**, a rapidly acting antianginal agent, is essentially ineffective when administered orally due to an extremely high first pass effect but is very effective in treating acute attacks of angina if given sublingually.

Transdermal patches and **ointment formulations** provide a continuous supply of drug over an extended period of time and are useful for rapidly metabolizing compounds such as nitroglycerin. These delivery systems, while not suited to treat acute anginal symptoms are effective in providing prophylactic concentrations of nitroglycerin.

Intramuscular depot injections also provide a continuous supply of drug over an extended period of time. Highly lipid soluble esters of **estradiol** and **testosterone** (e.g., Estradiol benzoate, testosterone enanthate) are slowly absorbed from their administration site. Hydrolysis of these Prodrugs produces a steady supply of these rapidly metabolized hormones.

Enteric-coated formulations can protect acid sensitive drugs as they pass through the acidic environment of the stomach. **Methamine, erythromycin**, and **omeprazole** are examples of acid sensitive agents that are available as enteric coated preparations.

Nasal administration allow for the delivery of peptides, such as **calcitonin salmon**, which have very low (if any) oral bioavailability. Characteristics of lung make it ideal for the administration of peptides. Aerosolized drugs only need to penetrate a thin epithelial layer to reach abundant capillary beds. Additionally the lungs contain protease inhibitors, which allow for greater stability of the peptides.

1.2.2. Pharmacological strategies involve the concurrent use of enzyme inhibitors to decrease drug metabolism. In some instances, the concurrent use of additional agent does not prevent the toxicity caused by metabolites of therapeutic agent[13].

Levodopa (L-dopa), the amino acid precursor of dopamine, is used in the treatment of Parkinsonism. Unlike dopamine, L-dopa can penetrate the blood brain barrier and reach the central nervous system. When in the brain, it is decarboxylated to dopamine. To ensure that adequate concentrations of L-dopa reach the CNS, peripheral metabolism of the drug must be blocked. The cocurrent administration of carbidopa, a dopa decarboxylase inhibitor that can not penetrate the blood brain barrier, prevents peripheral formation of dopamine and allows site specific delivery of dopamine to the CNS.

β-Lactam antibiotics. The antibacterial activity of a number of β-Lactam antibiotics is reduced by microorganisms capable of secreting the enzyme β-Lactamase. This enzyme hydrolyzes the β-Lactam ring and inactivates the antibiotic. To counter this resistance mechanism, a β-Lactamase inhibitor, such as clavulanic acid, is used in conjunction with penicillin, such as amoxycillin, to successfully treat infections caused by β-Lactamase-producing bacteria.

Ifosfamide is an alkylating agent that must undergo in vivo metabolism to produce active nitrogen mustard. In the process of this metabolic activation, significant concentration of acrolein is produced. These acrolein molecules react with nucleophiles on renal proteins and produce hemorrhagic cystitis. To prevent this toxicity, ifosfamide is always coadministered with mensa, a sulfhydryl containing compound that reacts with and neutralizes any acrolein that is present in the kidney.

HIV protease inhibitors are extensively metabolized by CYP3A isozymes. In addition, compounds within this class can inhibit these same isozymes. This latter action has been used to optimize therapy. Ritonavir is an HIV protease inhibitor that is known to cause hepatotoxicity at therapeutic doses. Lopinavir is an HIV protease inhibitor that is ineffective if used alone due to rapid CYP3A oxidation. A new strategy combines a low dose of ritonavir with a therapeutic dose of lopinavir. This results in an inhibition of CYP3A, the establishment of adequate plasma levels of lopinavir and therapeutic efficacy without hepatotoxicity.

1.2.3. Chemical strategies involve the addition, deletion, or isosteric modification of key functional groups. These molecular modifications hinder or completely eliminate metabolic transformations[13] (figure1.4)

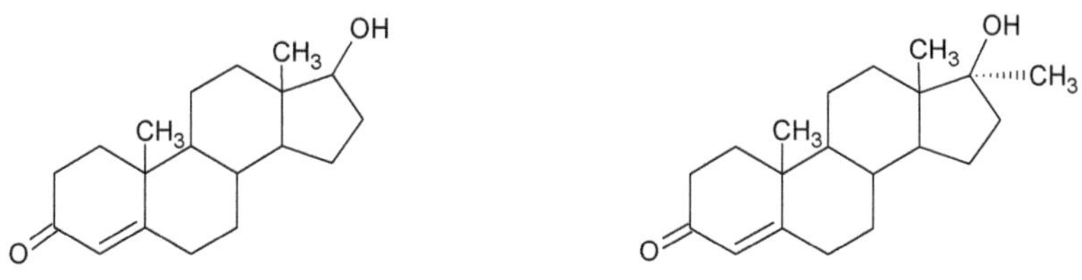

Testosterone Methyltestosterone

Figure1.4 Testosterone hydroxyl group is protected by methyl group from metabolism

Testosterone is not orally active due to rapid oxidation of its 17- hydroxyl group to a ketone. Addition of a 17α-methyl group converts the labile secondary alcohol to a stable tertiary alcohol. The resulting compound, Methyltestosterone, is only half as potent as testosterone; however it is not subject to rapid first pass metabolism and can be used orally. A similar strategy has been used to make orally active estradiol analogues.

Isoproterenol is a potent β-adrenergic agonist used for the relief of bronchospasm associated with bronchial asthma. Because it is cathecol (i.e., 3, 4-dihydroxy-substituted benzene ring), isoproterenol is subject to rapid metabolism by catechol O-methyl transferase (COMT) and thus has poor oral activity. Alteration of the 3, 4-dihydroxy substitution to a 3, 5-dihydroxy substitution produces metaproterenol, a bronchodilator that is not susceptible to COMT, is orally active, and has a longer duration of action than isoproterenol.

Octreotide is a synthetic octapeptide used to suppress or inhibit severe diarrhea associated with certain tumors. Octreotide mimics the actions of somatostatin, a naturally occurring 14-amino acid peptide. Somatostatin undergoes rapid proteolysis, has a half life of 1-3 minutes, and must be administered as a continuous intravenous infusion. Octreotide contains the amino acid essential for clinical efficacy but replaces two of the amino acids with their D-enantiomers. These unnatural D-amino acids are more resistant to hydrolysis. As a result, octreotide has an increased half life and can be administered as a subcutaneous injection.

There are various strategies that can be used to make drugs more resistant to hydrolysis and drug metabolism, and thus prolong their activity[14].

1.2.3.1 Steric shields

Some functional groups are more susceptible to chemical and enzymatic degradation than others. For example esters and amides are particularly prone to hydrolysis. A common strategy that is used to protect such groups is to add steric shields, designed to hinder the approach of a nucleophile or an enzyme to the susceptible group. These usually involve the addition of a bulky alkyl group close to the functional group. For example, the t-butyl group in the antirheumatic agent D1927 serves as steric shield and block hydrolysis of

terminal peptide bond (fig. 1.5)

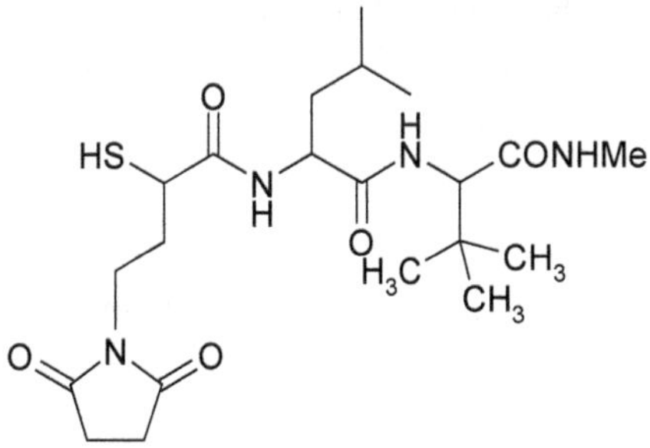

Stericshield

Figure1.5 The use of a steric shield to protect the antirheumatic agent D 1927

Steric shields have also been used to protect penicillins from Lactamases and to prevent drug interacting with cytochrome P450 enzymes.

1.2.3.2 Electronic effect of bioisosteres

Another popular tactic used to protect a labile functional group is to stabilize the group electronically using a bioisostere, a chemical group used to replace another chemical group within a drug, without affecting the important biological activity. Other features such as the drugs stability may also be improved. Isosteres and non classic isosteres are frequently used as bioisosteres. For example, replacing the methyl group of an ethanoate ester with an NH_2 result in a urethane functional group which is more stable than the original ester (fig. 1.6)

$$CH_3\text{-CO-O-R} \xrightarrow[\text{Isostere}]{} H_2N\text{-CO-O-R}$$

Figure 1.6 Isosteric replacement of a methyl group with an amino group

The NH_2 group is the same valency and size as the methyl group and therefore has no steric effect, but it has totally different electronic properties since it can feed electrons into the carboxyl group and stabilize it from hydrolysis. The cholinergic agonist **carbachol** is stabilized in this way, as is the cephalosporin **cefoxitin**.

$$H_2N\text{-}CO\text{-}O\text{-}CH_2\text{-}CH_2\text{-}\overset{+}{N}Me_3$$

Carbachol

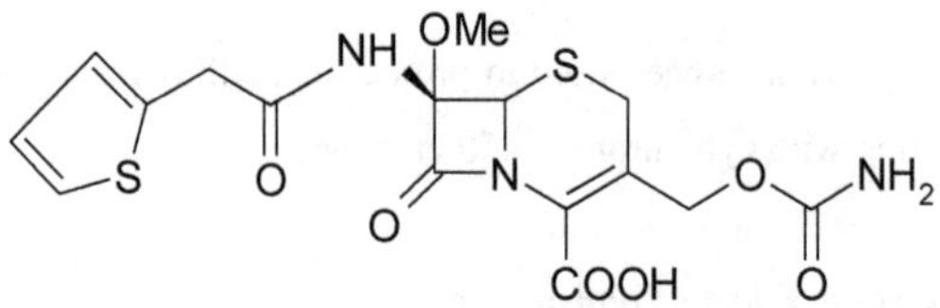

Cefoxitin

Alternatively, a labile ester group could be replaced by an amide group (NH replacing O). Amides are more resistant to chemical hydrolysis, due again to the lone pair of nitrogen feeding its electrons into the carbonyl group and making it less electrophilic.

It is important to realize that bioisosteres are not general and are often specific to a particular field. Replacing an ester with a urethane or an amide may work in one category of drugs but not another. One must also appreciate that bioisosteres are different from isosteres. It is the retention of important biological activity that determines whether a group is a bioisostere, not the valency. Therefore non isosteric group can be used as bioisosteres. For example, a pyrrole ring was used as a bioisostere for an amide bond in the development of the dopamine antagonist Du 122290 from sultopride.

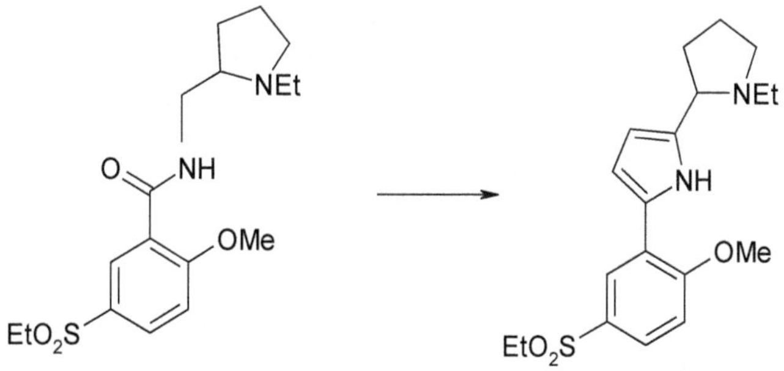

Sultopride DU 122290

Figure 1.7 Introducing a pyrrole ring as a bioisostere for an amide group.

Similarly, thiazoyl rings were used as bioisosteres for pyridine ring in the development of ritonavir.

One is not confined to the use of bioisosteres to increase stability. Groups or substituents having an inductive electronic effect have frequently been incorporated into molecules to increase the stability of a labile functional group. For example, electron withdrawing groups were incorporated into the side chain of penicillins to increase their resistance to acid hydrolysis. Because electron withdrawing group could draw electrons away from the carbonyl oxygen and reduce its tendency to act as a nucleophile (fig. 1.8)

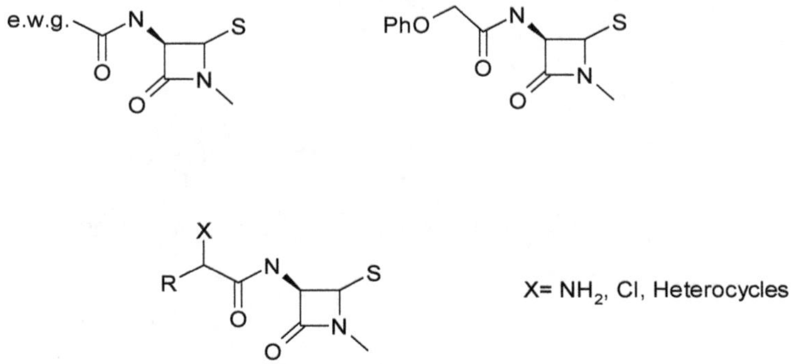

Figure1.8 Reduction of neighbouring group participation with an electron withdrawing group (e.w.g.)

1.2.3.3 Stereochemical modifications

Steric hindrance and electronic stabilization have often been used together to stabilize labile groups. For example, procaine (Fig. 1.9) is a good local anaesthetic, but it is short lasting because its ester group is quickly hydrolyzed. Changing the ester group to the less reactive amide group reduces chemical hydrolysis. Furthermore, the presence of two ortho- methyl groups on the aromatic ring helps to shield the carbonyl group from attack by nucleophiles or enzymes. This result in longer acting, local anaesthetic lidocaine. Since steric and electronic influences are both involved, the modifications are defined as stereoelectronic. Further successful examples of stereoelectronic modifications are demonstrated by oxacillin and bethanechol.

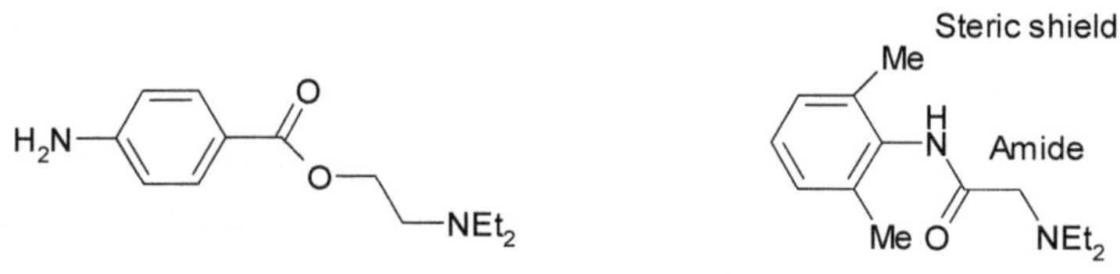

Procaine Lidocaine

Figure 1.9 Stereoelectronic modifications which make lidocaine a longer lasting, local anaesthetic compared with procaine

1.2.3.4 Metabolic blockers

Some drugs are metabolized by the introduction of polar groups at particular positions in their skeleton. For example, the oral contraceptive megesteol acetate is oxidized at position 6 to give a hydroxyl group at that position (Fig. 1.10). The introduction of polar hydroxyl group allows the formation of polar conjugates which can be quickly eliminated from the system. By introducing a methyl group at position 6, metabolism is blocked and the activity of the drug is prolonged[14].

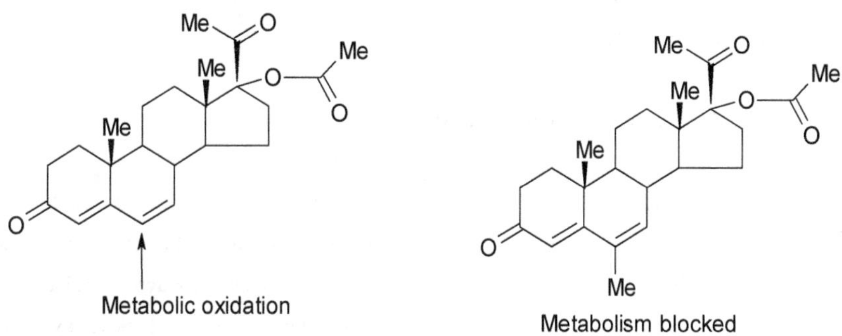

Megestrol acetate Analogue

Figure 1.10 Metabolic blocking by the addition of a methyl substituent

On the same lines, a popular method of protecting aromatic rings from metabolism at the para- position is to introduce a fluoro substituent. For example, CGP 52411 (Fig. 1.11) is an enzyme inhibitor which acts on the kinase active site of the epidermal growth factor receptor. It went forward for clinical trials as an anticancer agent and was found to undergo oxidative metabolism at the para position of the aromatic rings. Fluoro substituents were successfully added to block this metabolism and the analogue CGP 53353 was also put forward for clinical trials. This tactic was also applied successfully in the design of gefitinib.

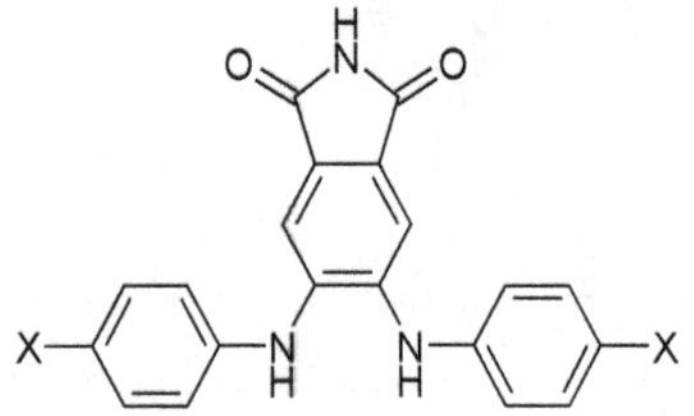

Figure 1.11 The use of fluorine substituents as metabolic blockers.

X = H, CGP 52411

X = OH, metabolite

X = F, CGP 53353

1.2.3.5 Removal or replacement of susceptible metabolic groups

Certain chemical groups are particularly susceptible to metabolic enzymes. For example, methyl groups on aromatic rings are often oxidized to carboxylic acids. These acids then are quickly eliminated from body. Other common metabolic reaction includes aliphatic and aromatic C-hydroxylation, N- and S-oxidations, O- and S-dealkylations, and deaminations[14].

Susceptible groups can sometimes be removed or replaced by groups that are stable to oxidation, in order to prolong the lifetime of the drug. For example, the aromatic methyl substituent of the antidiabetic Tolbutamide was replaced by a chloro substituent to give Chlorpropamide, which is much longer lasting (Fig. 1.12).

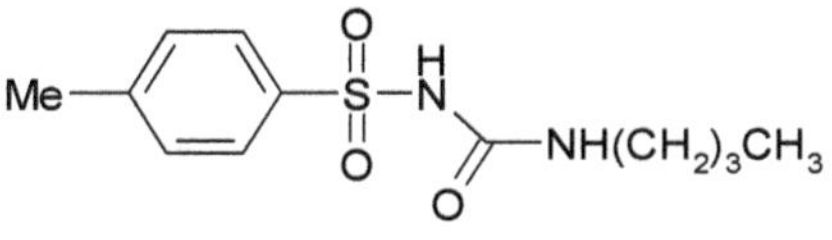

Tolbutamide

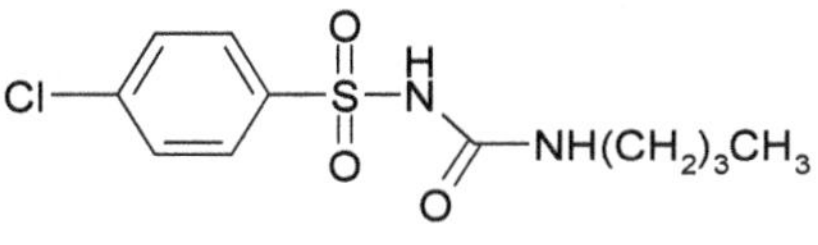

Chlorpropamide

Figure 1.12 Replacing metabolically labile groups

This tactic was also used in the design of gefitinib. An alternative strategy which is often tried is to replace the susceptible methyl group with CF_3, CHF_2 or CH_2F. The fluorine atoms alter the oxidation potential of the methyl group and make it more resistant to oxidation.

Another example, where a susceptible ester in cephalosporins is replaced with metabolically stable groups to give cephaloridine and cefalexin.

1.2.3.6 Group shifts

Removing or replacing a metabolically vulnerable group is feasible if the group concerned is not involved in important binding interactions with the binding site. If the group is important, then we have to use a different strategy.

There are two possible solutions. We can either mask the vulnerable group on a temporary basis by using a prodrug or we can try shifting the vulnerable group within the molecular skeleton. The latter tactic was used in the development of salbutamol (fig. 1.13)

Salbutamol was introduced in 1969 for the treatment of asthma, and is an analogue of the neurotransmitter noradrenaline- a catechol structure containing two ortho phenolic groups[14].

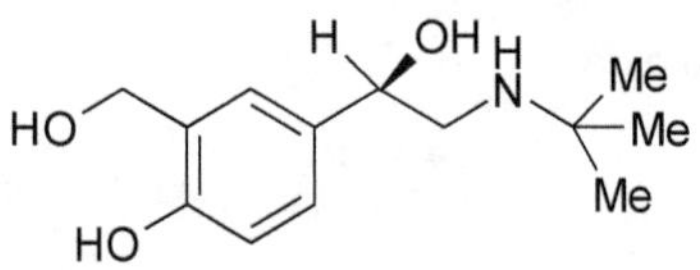

Salbutamol

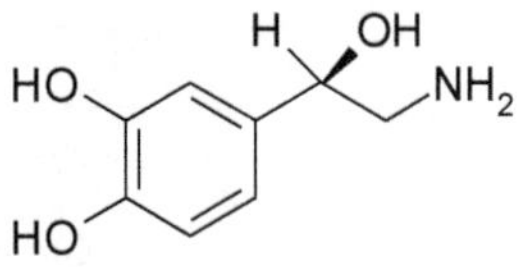

Noradrenaline

Figure 1.13 Salbutamol and noradrenaline

One of the problems faced by catechol compounds is metabolic methylation of one of the phenolic groups. Since both phenol groups are involved in hydrogen bonds to the receptor, methylation of one of the phenol groups disrupts the hydrogen bonding and makes the compound inactive. For example, the noradrenaline analogue (I in Fig. 1.14) has useful anti asthmatic activity, but the effect is of short duration because the compound is rapidly metabolized to the inactive methyl ether (II in Fig. 1.14)

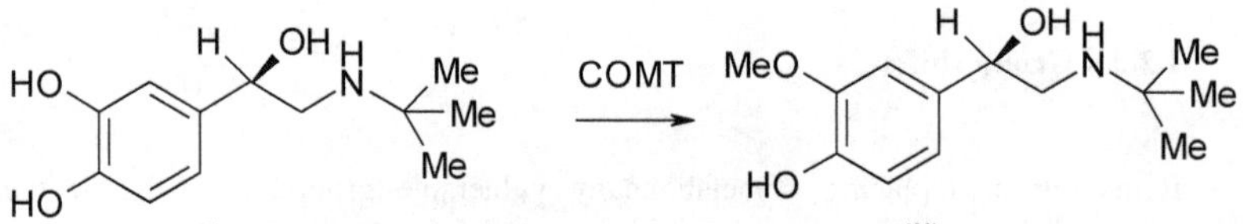

Figure 1.14 Metabolic methylation of a noradrenaline analogue

Removing the OH or replacing it with a methyl group prevents metabolism, but also prevents the important hydrogen bonding interactions with the binding site. Solution of this problem was to move the vulnerable hydroxyl group out from the ring by one carbon unit. This was enough to make the compound unrecognizable to the metabolic enzyme but not to the receptor binding site.

Fortunately, the receptor appears to be quite lenient over the position of this hydrogen bonding group and it is interesting to note that a hydroxyethyl group is also acceptable. Beyond that, activity is lost because the OH group is out of range, or too large to fit. These results demonstrate that it is better to consider a binding region within the receptor binding site as an available volume, rather than imagining it as being fixed at one spot. A drug can then be designed such that the relevant binding group is positioned into any part of that available volume.

Shifting an important binding but metabolically susceptible group worked for salbutamol, but one cannot guarantee that the same tactic will always be successful. Shifting the group may make the molecule unrecognizable both to its target and to the metabolic enzyme.

1.2.3.7 Ring variation and ring substituents

Certain ring systems may be susceptible to metabolism, and so varying the ring might improve metabolic stability. This can be done by adding nitrogen into the ring to lower the electron density of the ring system. For example, the imidazole ring of the antifungal agent tioconazole is susceptible to metabolism, but replacement with a 1, 2, 4-triazole ring as in fluconazole results in improved stability[14] (Fig. 1.15)

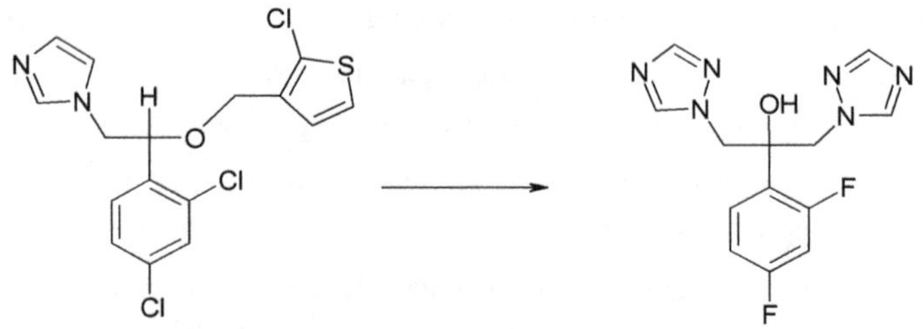

Ticonazole Fluconazole

Figure 1.15 Increasing stability in antifungal agent

Electron rich aromatic rings such as phenyl groups are particularly prone to oxidative metabolism, but can be stabilized by replacing them with nitrogen containing heterocyclic rings such as pyridine or pyrimidine. Alternatively, electron withdrawing substituents could be added to the aromatic ring to lower the electron density.

Ring variation can also help to stabilize metabolically susceptible aromatic or heteroaromatic methyl substituents. Such substituents could be replaced with more stable substituents, but sometimes the methyl substituent is to be retained for good activity. In such cases, introducing a nitrogen atom into the aromatic/heteroaromatic ring can be beneficial, since lowering the electron density in the ring also helps to make the methyl substituent more resistant to metabolism. For example, F13640 is undergoing phase II clinical trials as an analgesic (Fig. 1.16).

The methyl substituent on the pyridine ring is susceptible to oxidation and is converted to carboxylic acid which is inactive. The methyl group plays an important binding role and has to be present. Therefore the pyridine ring was changed to a pyrimidine ring resulting in a compound (F15599) that has increased metabolic stability without affecting binding affinity.

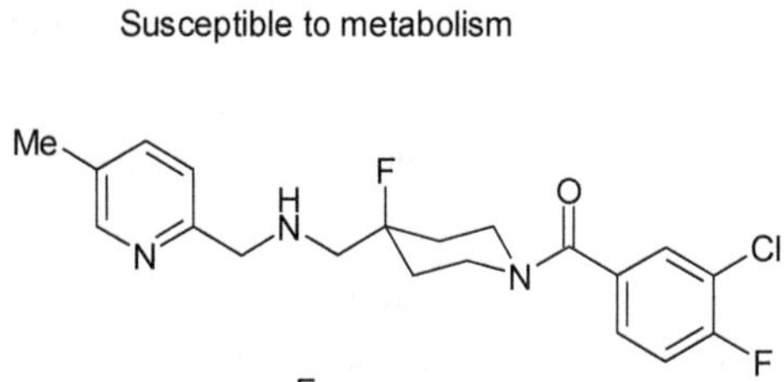

F_{13640}

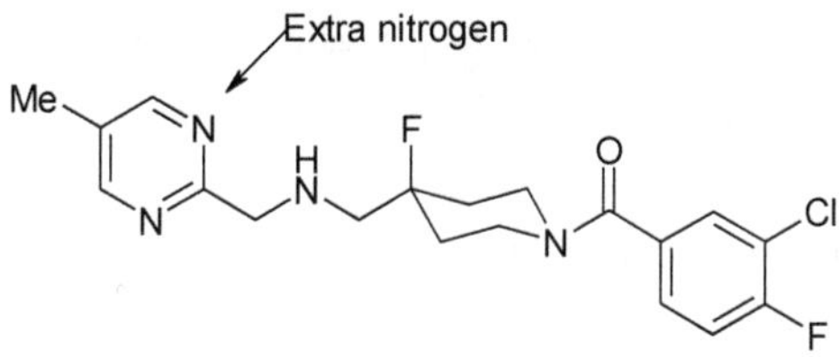

F_{15599}

Figure 1.16 Stabilizing an aromatic or heteroaromatic methyl substituent by adding a nitrogen to the ring

1.3 DRUG DELIVERY SYSTEMS (DDS) FOR ENHANCING HALF-LIFE

DDS are classified as a function of the structure and the release mechanism into: (a) membrane based systems, where the drug is dispersed inside of a polymer membrane and the release can be controlled by drug diffusion or by osmotic pressure, (b) matrix based systems, where the drug is dispersed in a polymeric matrix and its release can be controlled by drug diffusion or matrix erosion,(c) hydrophilic matrices where the drug release is controlled either by matrix swelling or by the matrix slow dissolution, (d) stimuli responsive systems where drug release is controlled by changes in stimuli such as temperature or pH, and (e), polymer-drug conjugates where drug release is chemically controlled.

Covalent polymer-drug conjugates are a special type of DDS where the drug or bioactive compound (peptides, proteins, growth factors, hormones, enzymes, etc.) is covalently linked to the macromolecular backbone through a physiologically labile bond[15]. The possibility of linking any bioactive molecule to a macromolecular chain makes polymeric conjugated systems very useful for applications not only related to medication, but also in fields as tissue engineering, biosensors, affinity separations, enzymatic processes, cell culture, etc.

1.3.1 Synthetic polymer-drug conjugates (the ringsdorf model)

The concept of covalent polymer-drug conjugates was firstly introduced by Helmut Ringsdorf in 1975, who called them synthetic polymeric drugs or pharmacologically active polymers[16]. His model is based on the covalent link between the drug and a macromolecular backbone through a labile bond.

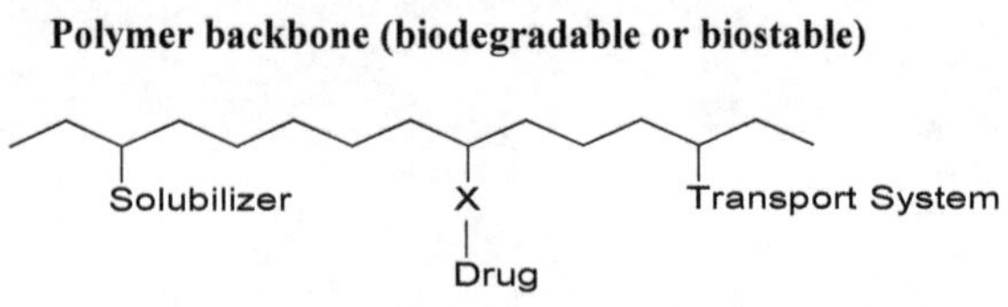

Figure 1.17 Ringsdorf model of synthetic polymer drugs.

Figure 1.17 shows the scheme of the Ringsdorf model where a biostable or biodegradable polymer backbone carries three different units. A hydrophilic area used to make the whole macromolecule soluble and non-toxic, a second region in which the drug is linked to the polymer chain, and a third area that incorporates a transport system whose function is to carry the whole polymer to the target cells or site of pharmacological action. The separation of the different areas along the macromolecular chain may be accomplished by statistical terpolymerization or block copolymerization.

In addition, polymer properties can be induced by the polymer specific structural characteristics such as high molecular weight, coil structure, neighbouring groups' effects, copolymer composition, variable polyelectrolyte charges, flexibility of polymer chains, and microstructure. In this sense, the advantages of this type of DDS are their diversity in composition, molecular structure and molecular weight, being predominantly used hydrophilic systems with polar or ionic groups, which lead to polymer water solubility and reactivity for conjugation with bioactive molecules. The different ways that can be used to chemically link the bioactive molecules to the polymer chains by hydrolysable or biodegradable bonds are multiple and are shown in Figure 18. As it will be discussed below, the reactive groups can be linked at the end of the polymer chain (end groups), or in the side chain (pendant groups).

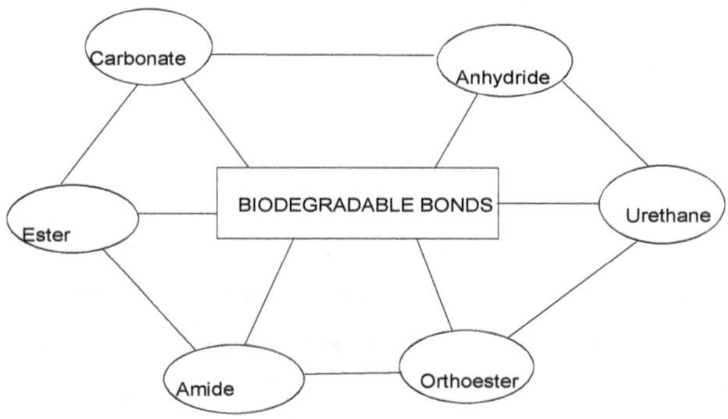

Figure 1.18 Biodegradable bonds used to conjugate bioactive molecules to polymer backbones.

Other important aspects that are also some limitations of the synthetic polymers used in this type of applications are: a) non-toxic and non-immunogenic, b) clearable from the body without any accumulations in tissues or organs, c) controlled average molecular weight and molecular weight distribution avoiding undesirable responses of low or high Mw polymer-drug conjugates, d) high purity of polymers, e) possible sterilization of polymers with biodegradable character.

These types of DDSs are probably the most attractive devices because they are designed on the molecular basis. However, in despite of the high versatility of this approach, it is difficult to find marketed products mainly because these conjugates are considered as new drug molecules and the path needed to be approved is arduous and expensive.

The three areas of the Ringsdorf model exposed in Figure 1.17 provide the different possibilities from the chemical point of view to design and prepare covalent polymer-drug conjugates with specific applications. The most important requirement of the solubilizer area is to provide non-toxic and non-immunogenic character, as well as to give a soluble character to the polymer chain. Water solubilizing units have generally been introduced with co-monomers such as vinyl pyrrolidone (VP) or acrylamides, whereas in the case of lipid-solubilizing units co-monomers bearing alkyl side chains Increase the possible absorption at lipid phases and cell membranes. As mentioned above, the polymer molecular weight and molecular weight distribution are significant as soluble polymers can be excreted via the glomerular kidney membrane which are below 50,000 Da.

The second area of Figure 1.17 is that of the drug bonded to the polymer chain, where aspects as fixing the drug in mild conditions, the nature of the chemical fixing groups (see Figure 1.18), and the nature of the drug are of great interest when designing this type of DDS. The drug fixation must be mild enough to allow attachment without any adverse effect on its biological activity. In this sense, polymerizable active esters and amides have been widely used. Connected to this area is the release of the drug and its relationship with the spacer groups between the polymer and the drug. The drug might be required to be released fast or slow and the release rate can be modulated by the type of the spacer group. A permanent spacer separates the drug from the polymer backbone, and interferes to the biological activity of the bound material, being an example the direct fixation of enzymes which leads to loss its enzymatic activity when directly bonded to the polymer, activity which is restored when the enzyme is attached through a long alkyl group. Temporary spacer groups are a type of spacers applied to release the active molecule. A typical example is the presence of peptides groups bounded to the polymer chain and to the drug[17].

The third area of Figure 1.17 is the transport system which function is to induce specific or non-specific resorption at the target cells or local site of pharmacological activity. Specific resorption at the biological target can be achieved by using homing devices, i.e. receptor-active components like immunoglobulin, enzymes, hormones or special drugs, as it has been demonstrated in cancer chemotherapy[16]. On the other hand, non-specific resorption enhancers can be produced by inducing variations in the normal body distribution of polymers that can be expected in surface, membrane and skin active systems with, for example, sulfoxides or formamide groups which enhance the uptake of certain drugs through the skin. Other special type of transport systems are those based on the fixation via reactive esters that can be obtained by local injections into specific areas (tumours or tissues), or by simply fixation of the reactive ester to the intestinal wall.

Types of polymer-drug conjugates

The classification of this type of DDS is based on the conjugation sites of the mentioned reactive groups. These reactive groups can be used for conjugations via end groups or pendant polymer groups. In the pendant polymer groups the same or different biomolecules can be conjugated to a given polymer chain by controlling the number of the reactive pendant groups, including spacers between them and the bioactive molecule and maintaining the biodegradable character of the links, whereas in the polymer end group model, the conjugation only can be produced in one or two extremes of the chain ends.

Despite the great versatility in composition, structure and molecular weight of synthetic polymers, one of the simplest polymers, polyethylene glycol, PEG, has been the most widely used in end group synthetic polymer-biomolecule conjugates. This approach has found an important application in the so-called protein PEGylation (see Figure 19), based on the conjugation of the PEG to protein drugs to protect them from recognition by the immune body system, and to prolong their circulation time in the body, as described by Abuchowski *et al.* in 1977 about the alterations of immunological properties of bovine serum albumin (BSA), covalently attached to PEG[18]. All the modifications on PEG have been based on the replacement of the hydroxyl end group, also taken into consideration the influence of the molecular weight of the PEG chains and the site of conjugation, that influence the final properties of the conjugates[19]. In this sense, PEG with average molecular weight of several thousands have generally been used, and the majority of the PEG-protein conjugations have been performed via the lysine amino group of the protein, although other reactive sites of histidine and cysteine can be employed[20]. Other type of conjugation developed with PEG are some interesting branched, star and comb-like polymers that have been conjugated with proteins[21].

Figure 1.19 Typical end-group polymer-drug conjugate based on polyethylene glycol (PEG) modifications.

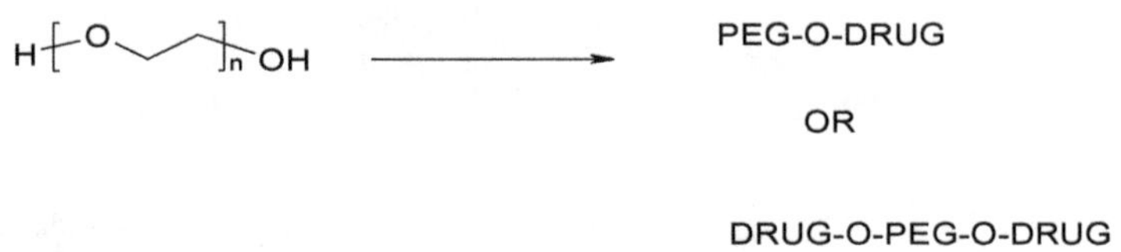

Many efforts have been made to achieve an efficient and stable coupling of PEG chains to the biopharmaceutical. Very successful developments have been achieved with regard to the variability of the coupling chemistry and the availability of specialized linkers[22].

Site-specific monoPEGylation is of significant relevance in order to provide highly reproducible products maintaining maximum activity. In the majority of cases, high molecular weight PEG chains (10 – 40kDa) are used for the monoPEGylation of proteins. At best, it is possible to attach one single PEG chain to the N-terminal amino group of a protein by reductive amination. Especially with small proteins, such as cytokines, it is possible to apply genetic methods to introduce rare amino acids, which then can be used for the coupling of PEG[23]. Preferred for this purpose is a cystein residue which can be specifically PEGylated at the thiol group by maleimide coupling. Some examples have also been published in which the site-directed PEGylation has been achieved by an enzyme catalyzed reaction with a transglutaminase[24].

Branched PEG reagents showed superior protecting properties compared with linear molecules.Today there are only a few commercial examples of such branched PEG molecules, because very often their synthesis is complex and time-consuming. However, some important progress in this field is expected in the next few years.

Meanwhile, there are some successful commercial examples of PEGylated drugs. Many others are under clinical development or close to approval. The first ever PEGylated drug on the market was ADAGEN® (PEGylated Adenosine deaminase), produced by Enzon, which is used for the treatment of a severe combined immune deficiency in children and adolescents (SCID-disease), caused mainly by the lack of the body's own Adenosine deaminase. ADAGEN® was approved under the orphan drug act in 1990 on the basis of a clinical trial with 6 patients. This method of therapy, called enzyme replacement therapy, is the starting point for the treatment of many genetically caused diseases of the metabolism[25]. The market success of such an enzyme drug for human therapy very often heavily depends on an efficient PEGylation.

A further established PEGylated enzyme drug is, for example, PEG-Aspargase (ONCASPAR®) for the treatment of acute lymphoblastic leukemia in children. The major advantage of ONCASPAR®is a prolonged plasma half-life and a strongly reduced immunogenicity compared to the nonPEGylated Asparaginase. Other PEGylated enzymes to be mentioned are Uricase, Glutaminase,Arginine deiminase and Glucocerebrosidase. These drugs are still under clinical development.

Cytokines are commercially the most important biopharmaceuticals today. Even their efficiency has been improved by PEGylation. Blockbuster products are PEG-α-Interferon 2b (PEG-INTRON) and PEG-α-Interferon 2a (PEGASYS) [26], which are used for the treatment of infections with hepatitis C virus. Both proteins have a very similar amino acid sequence, however they may be distinguished by the kind of PEG chains used for PEGylation. PEG-INTRON has been conjugated with a linear PEG molecule with a molecular weight of 10 kDa, while PEGASYS has been modified with a branched reagent consisting of two 20kDa PEG chains. PEGASYS is superior to PEG-INTRON because of a higher specific activity and a prolonged plasma half-life.

After two decades of experience, PEGylation technology can be regarded as a proved and tested method for the drug delivery of biopharmaceuticals, especially proteins. Already today, biopharmaceuticals are a multibillion-dollar market which is expected to grow rapidly within the next decade. The sales of several PEGylated drugs such as PEG-INTRON have reached 3 billion US $, comparable to the sales of conventional synthetic blockbusters. However, the development of PEG technology is by no means finished. Recent publications reveal that some questions still remain to be resolved. In particular, there is a requirement for new synthetic routes to provide functionally expanded PEG reagents of reproducible high quality. Site-specific conjugation will be one of the major topics for the coming years, especially with regard to technically applicable and commercially reasonable solutions.

Many investigations are under way to explore new fields for the application of PEGylation. These are manifold and not limited to protein drugs or biopharmaceuticals. In the area of oncology, for example, the coupling of conventional synthetic drugs (so-called "small molecules"), such as Ara-C[27] or Camptothecin[28], to polymers resulted in a significant reduction of toxicity and an increased selectivity for tumour tissue. The latter phenomenon is based on a nonspecific accumulation of large molecules in malignant tissue. This effect is called the EPR effect: enhanced permeability and retention. Other promising applications for PEGylation are PEGylation of liposomes, nonviral gene shuttles, nanoparticles, oligonucleotides and surfaces for technical or medical devices[29].

Due to the increasing relevance of biopharmaceuticals and the high regulatory demands for their approval, innovative and specialized drug delivery systems have gained considerable importance.Thus, intelligent drug delivery systems such as PEGylation will determine the commercial success of the pharmaceutical industry in the future. With its broad applicability, high efficiency and comparably low costs, PEGylation will maintain a leading position. As a result, PEGylation, alone or in combination with other drug delivery technologies, will be an essential part of a successful strategy for the development of biopharmaceutical drugs.

In a nut shell main advantages of biomolecules conjugated with PEG (PEGylation) are based on the following aspects:

a) PEG is essentially non-toxic (approved for human use)

b) Is easily activated for conjugation and inexpensive

c) Conjugates have improved solubility and stability

d) Posses higher resistance to surface adsorption

e) Exhibit prolonged circulation time in the bloodstream due to increase in the hydrodynamic size (size in solution) of the agent

f) Reduced dosage frequency, without diminished efficacy with potentially reduced toxicity

g) Have reduced immunogenicity and antigenicity because covalent attachment of PEG to a drug or therapeutic protein can mask the agent from the host's immune system.

h) Have controlled permeability through biological barriers.

i) Increased bioavailability

One of the most important limitations is that many different sites of the protein may be conjugated to the polymer molecules, interfering sometimes with the active recognition pocket and reducing the bioactivity of the protein[30]. Despite this aspect, there are many examples in the literature of increase biological activity of biomolecules after their end group conjugation to polymer macromolecules[31].

1.3.2 Dendrimer as drug carrier

Nanoparticle drug-delivery systems are the popular ones as are able to increase the selectivity and stability of therapeutic agents. However reticuloendothelial system (RES) uptake, drug leakage, immunogenicity, hemolytic toxicity, cytotoxicity, hydrophobicity restrict the use of these nanostructures. These shortcomings are overcome by surface engineering the dendrimer such as Polyester dendrimer, Citric acid dendrimer, Arginine dendrimer, Glycodendrimers, PEGylated dendrimers, etc. The bioactive agents can be easily encapsulated into the interior of the dendrimers or chemically attached i.e. conjugated or physically adsorbed onto the dendrimer surface, serving the desired properties of the carrier to the specific needs of the active material and its therapeutic applications. In addition to supplying a multivalent backbone for drug attachment, dendrimers also provide access to various new polymer architectures that are potentially relevant to drug delivery applications.

A. Description[32, 33, 34]

A dendrimer is generally described as a macromolecule, which is characterized by its highly branched 3D structure that provides a high degree of surface functionality and versatility. Dendrimers have often been referred to as the "Polymers of the 21st century". Dendrimer chemistry was first introduced in 1978 by Fritz Vogtle and coworkers. He synthesized the first "cascade molecules". In 1985, Donald A. Tomalia, synthesized the first family of dendrimers. The word "*dendrimer*" originated from two words, the Greek word *dendron*, meaning tree, and *meros*, meaning part. At the same time, Newkome's group independently reported synthesis of similar macromolecules. They called them *arborols* from the Latin word 'arbor' also meaning a tree. The term *cascade molecule* is also used, but 'dendrimer' is the best established one. Due to their multivalent and monodisperse character, dendrimers have stimulated wide interest in the field of chemistry and biology, especially in applications like drug delivery, gene therapy and chemotherapy.

B. Structure [35, 36, 37]

Dendrimers are built from a starting atom, such as nitrogen, to which carbon and other elements are added by a repeating series of chemical reactions that produce a spherical branching structure. As the process repeats, successive layers are added, and the sphere can be expanded to the size required by the investigator. The result is a spherical macromolecular structure whose size is similar to albumin and hemoglobin, but smaller than such multimers as the gigantic IgM antibody complex.

Dendrimers possess three distinguished architectural components, namely

(i) An initiator core.

(ii) Interior layers (generations) composed of repeating units, radically attached to the interior core.

(iii) Exterior (terminal functionality) attached to the outermost interior generations.

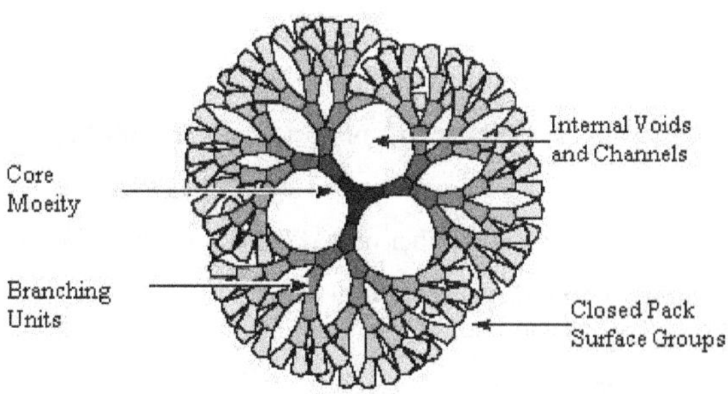

Figure 1.20: The Dendritic Structure

Components of a Dendrimer Structure

Generation

It is the hyperbranching when going from the centre of the dendrimer towards the periphery, resulting in homostructural layers between the focal points (branching points). The number of focal points when going from the core towards the dendrimer surface is the generation number. That is a dendrimer having five focal points when going from the centre to the periphery is denoted as the 5th generation dendrimer. Here, we abbreviate this term to simply a G5-dendrimer, *e.g.* a 5th generation polypropylene imine is abbreviated to a "G5-PPI-" dendrimer, The core part of the dendrimer is sometimes denoted generation "zero", or in the terminology presented here "G0". The core structure thus presents no focal points, as hydrogen substituents are not considered focal points. Intermediates during the dendrimer synthesis are sometimes denoted half-generations; a well-known example is the carboxylic acid-terminated Poly (amidoamine) dendrimers (PAMAM) dendrimers.

Shell

The dendrimer shell is the homo-structural spatial segment between the focal points, the "generation space". The "outer shell" is the space between the last outer branching point and the surface. The "inner shells" are generally referred to as the dendrimer interior.

Pincer

In dendrimers, the outer shell consists of a varying number of pincers created by the last focal point before reaching the dendrimer surface. In PPI and PAMAM dendrimers the number of pincers is half the number of surface groups (because in these dendrimers the chain divides into two chains in each focal point).

End-group

It is also generally referred to as the "terminal group" or the "surface group" of the dendrimer. Dendrimers having amine end-groups are termed "amino-terminated dendrimers".

Types of Dendrimers [35,38,39,40]

Pamam Dendrimer

Poly (amidoamine) dendrimers (PAMAM) are synthesized by the divergent method starting from ammonia or ethylenediamine initiator core reagents. Products up to generation 10[(7)] (a molecular weight of over 9, 30,000 g/mol) have been obtained (by comparison, the molecular weight of human hemoglobin is approximately 65,000 g/mol). PAMAM dendrimers are commercially available, usually as methanol solutions. *Starburst dendrimers* is applied as a trademark name for a sub-class of PAMAM dendrimers based on a tris-aminoethylene-imine core. The name refers to the star like pattern observed when looking at the structure of the high-generation dendrimers of this type in two-dimensions.

Pamamos Dendrimer

Radially layered poly (amidoamine-organosilicon) dendrimers (PAMAMOS) are inverted unimolecular micelles that consist of hydrophilic, nucleophilic polyamidoamine (PAMAM) interiors and hydrophobic organosilicon (OS) exteriors. These dendrimers are exceptionally useful precursors for the preparation of honeycomb-like networks with nanoscopic PAMAM and OS domains.

PPI Dendrimer

PPI-dendrimers stand for "Poly (Propylene Imine)" describing the propylamine spacer moieties in the oldest known dendrimer type developed initially by Vögtle. These dendrimers are generally poly-alkyl amines having primary amines as end groups, the dendrimer interior consists of numerous of tertiary tris-propylene amines. PPI dendrimers are commercially available up to G5, and has found widespread applications in material science as well as in biology. As an alternative name to PPI, POPAM is sometimes used to describe this class of dendrimers. POPAM stands for Poly (Propylene Amine), which closely resembles the PPI abbreviation. In addition, these dendrimers are also sometimes denoted "DAB-dendrimers" where DAB refers to the core structure, which is usually based on Diamino butane.

Tecto Dendrimer

These are composed of a core dendrimer, surrounded by dendrimers of several steps (each type design) to perform a function necessary for a smart therapeutic nanodevice. Different compounds perform varied functions ranging from diseased cell recognition, diagnosis of disease state drug delivery, reporting location to reporting outcomes of therapy.

Multilingual Dendrimers

In these dendrimers, the surface contains multiple copies of a particular functional group.

Chiral Dendrimers

The chirality in these dendrimers is based upon the construction of constitutionally different but chemically similar branches to chiral core.

Hybrid Dendrimers Linear Polymers

These are hybrids (block or graft polymers) of dendritic and linear polymers.

Amphiphilic Dendrimers

They are built with two segregated sites of chain end, one half is electron donating and the other half is electron withdrawing.

Micellar Dendrimers

These are unimolecular micelles of water soluble hyper branched polyphenylenes.

Multiple Antigen Peptide Dendrimers

It is a dendron-like molecular construct based upon a polylysine skeleton. Lysine with its alkyl amino side-chain serves as a good monomer for the introduction of numerous of branching points. This type of dendrimer was introduced by J. P. Tam in 1988, has predominantly found its use in biological applications, *e.g.* vaccine and diagnostic research.

Fréchet-Type Dendrimers

It is a more recent type of dendrimer developed by Hawker and Fréchet based on poly-benzyl ether hyper branched skeleton. These dendrimers usually have carboxylic acid groups as surface groups, serving as a good anchoring point for further surface functionalisation, and as polar surface groups to increase the solubility of this hydrophobic dendrimer type in polar solvents or aqueous media.

C. Syntheses [41, 43, 44]

The syntheses used for dendrimer preparation permit almost entire control over the critical molecular design parameters such as size, shape, surface/interior chemistry, flexibility, and topology. Many dendrimer syntheses rely upon traditional reactions, such as the Michael reaction or the Williamson ether synthesis whilst others involve the use of modern techniques and chemistry, such as solid-phase synthesis, organo-transition-metal chemistry, organosilicon chemistry, organo-phosphorus chemistry, or other contemporary organic methodologies. The choice of the growth reaction dictates the way in which the branching should be introduced into the dendrimer. Branching may either be present in the building blocks as is more often the case or it can be created as a function of the growth reaction, as is the case with the poly (amidoamine)s and the poly (propylene imine)s .

'Divergent' Dendrimer Growth [41, 44]

The synthetic methodology employed in the early dendrimer syntheses came to be known as the 'divergent' approach. This name comes from the way in which the dendrimer grows outwards from the core, diverging into space. Starting from a reactive core, a generation is grown, and then the new periphery of the molecule is activated for reaction with more monomers. The two steps can be repeated. The divergent approach is successful for the production of large quantities of dendrimers since, in each generation-adding step, the molar mass of the dendrimer is doubled. Divergently grown dendrimers are virtually impossible to isolate pure from their side products. The synthetic chemist must rely on extremely efficient reactions in order to ensure low polydispersities. The first synthesized dendrimers were **polyamidoamines (PAMAMs)**.They are also known as *starbust dendrimers* .Ammonia is used as the core molecule & In the presence of methanol, it reacts with methylacrylate and then ethylenediamine is added: [44]

$$NH_3 + 3CH_2CHCOOCH_3 \rightarrow \mathbf{N\,(CH_2\,CH_2COOCH_3)_3}$$

$$3\,NH_2\,CH_2\,CH_2NH_2 + \mathbf{N\,(CH_2\,CH_2COOCH_3)_3} \rightarrow N\,(CH_2\,CH_2CONHCH_2\,CH_2NH_2)_3 + 3CH_3OH$$

At the end of each branch there is a free amino group that can react with 2 methyl acrylate monomers and 2 ethylenediamine molecules. Each complete reaction sequence results in a new dendrimer generation. The number of reactive surface sites is doubled with every generation the mass increases more than twice [41].

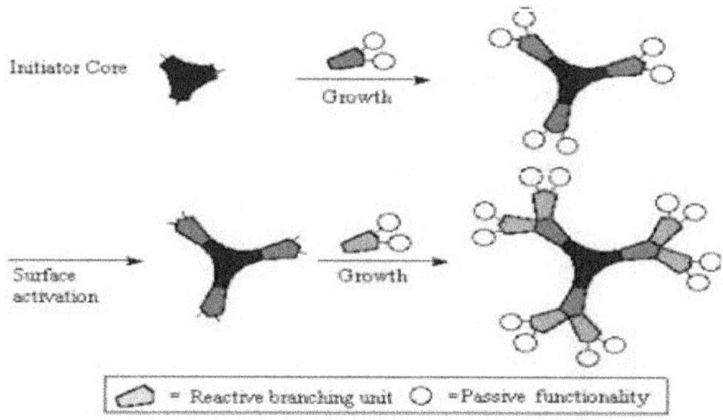

Figure 1.21: Divergent Dendrimer Growth

'Convergent' Dendrimer Growth [41, 44]

The 'convergent' approach was developed as a response to the weaknesses of divergent syntheses. Convergent growth begins at what will end up being the surface of the dendrimer, and works inwards by gradually linking surface units together with more. When the growing wedges are large enough, several units are attached to a suitable core to give a complete dendrimer. The advantages of convergent growth over divergent growth stem are that only two simultaneous reactions are required for any generation-adding step [36]. The convergent methodology also suffers from low yields in the synthesis of large structures. The convergent growth method has several advantages:

1. Relatively easy to purify the desired product and the occurrence of defects in the final structure is minimized.

2. Possible to introduce subtle engineering into the dendritic structure by precise placement of functional groups at the periphery of the macromolecules.

3. Approach does not allow the formation of high generation dendrimer because steric problems occur in the reactions of the dendrons and the core molecule [33].

D. Properties of Dendrimers [35, 42, 46-67]

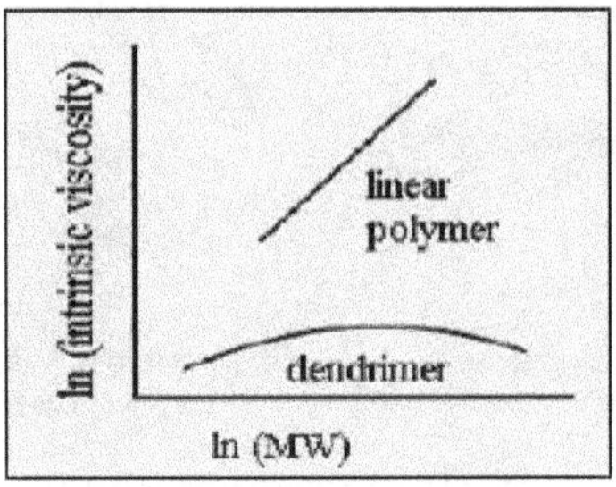

Figure 1.22: Correlation between intrinsic viscosity and Molecular weight

The classical polymerization process, which results in linear polymers, is usually random in nature and produces molecules of different sizes, whereas size and molecular mass of dendrimers can be specifically controlled during synthesis. Dendrimers are monodisperse macromolecules, unlike linear polymers. Because of their molecular architecture, dendrimers show some significantly improved physical and chemical properties when compared to traditional linear polymers. In solution, linear chains exist as flexible coils; in contrast, dendrimers form a tightly packed ball. This has a great impact on their rheological properties. Lower generation dendrimers, which are large enough to be spherical but do not form a tightly packed surface, have enormous surface areas in relation to volume. In contrast to linear polymers the intrinsic viscosity of dendrimer solutions does not increase linearly with mass but shows a maximum at a specific generation and then begins to decline [42,46]. Such behaviors are unlike that of linear polymers. This is likely to be because of the way in which dendrimer shape changes with generation, i.e. lower generations adopt a more open planar–elliptical shape with transition to a more compact spherical shape for higher generations. The presence of many chain ends is responsible for high solubility and miscibility and for high reactivity. In the structure of dendrimer (Fig. 1.23) the molecular density is theoretically highest in the periphery of the dendrimers. It has been suggested that back folding of the terminal branches leads to a more uniform or even reverse density profile [47] (Fig. 1.23). In nature tree-like structures have evolved to maximize the exposed surface area, e.g. to maximize the light exposure/number of leaves of a tree. In a similar fashion dendritic architecture creates molecules where a large proportion of the groups are exposed at the surface and which can have very high molecular surface to volume ratios (up to 1000 m^2/g). The presence of numerous terminal groups in dendrimers facilitates multiple simultaneous interactions of surface groups with the solvent, surfaces or other molecules and, as a consequence, dendrimers tend to show high solubility, reactivity, and binding.

Table 1.2: Properties of Dendrimer and linear polymers

Sr. No.	Property	Dendrimers	Linear Polymers
1	Structure	Compact, Globular	Not compact
2	Synthesis	Careful & stepwise growth	Single step polycondensation
3	Structural control	Very high	Low
4	Architecture	Regular	Irregular
5	Shape	Spherical	Random coil
6	Crystallanity	Non-crystalline, amorphous materials -lower glass temperatures	Semi crystalline/crystalline materials -Higher glass temperatures
7	Aqueous solubility	High	Low
8	Nonpolar solubility	High	Low
9	Viscosity	Non linear relationship with molecular weight	Linear relation with molecular weight
10	Reactivity	High	Low
11	Compressibility	Low	High
12	Polydispersity	Monodisperse	Polydisperse

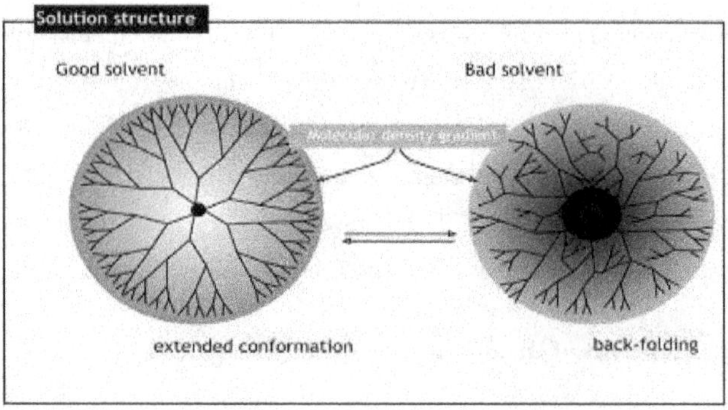

Figure 1.23: Dendrimer conformation.

This multivalency is of particular importance for biomedical applications. The multiple interactions between surface amines and nucleic aid phosphates are also important for the formation of dendrimers and DNA complexes. Dendrimers' solubility is strongly influenced by the nature of surface groups. Dendrimers terminated in hydrophilic groups are soluble in polar solvents, while dendrimers having hydrophobic end groups are soluble in nonpolar solvents. In a solubility test with tetrahydrofuran (THF) as the solvent, the solubility of dendritic polyester was found remarkably higher than that of analogous linear polyester. A marked difference was also observed in chemical reactivity.

Effect of Various Factors on the Properties of Dendrimers [48, 49]

Effect Of pH

Amino-terminated PPI and PAMAM dendrimers [48] have basic surface groups as well as a basic interior. For these types of dendrimers with interiors containing tertiary amines, the low pH region generally leads to extended conformations due to electrostatic repulsion between the positively charged ammonium groups. Applying molecular dynamics to predict the structural behaviour of PAMAM dendrimers as a function of pH show that the dendrimer has an extended conformation, based on a highly ordered structure at low pH (pH<4). At this pH, the interior is getting increasingly "hollow" as the generation number increases as a result of repulsion between the positively charged amines both at the dendrimer surface and the tertiary amines in the interior. At neutral pH, back-folding occurs which may be a consequence of hydrogen bonding between the uncharged tertiary amines in the interior and the positively charged surface amines. At higher pH (pH>10) the dendrimer contracts as the charge of the molecule becomes neutral, acquiring a more spherical (globular) structure, where the repulsive forces between the dendrimer arms and between the surface groups reaches a minimum. At this pH, the conformation has a higher degree of back-folding as a consequence of the weak "inter-dendron" repulsive forces (Figure 1.24).[49]

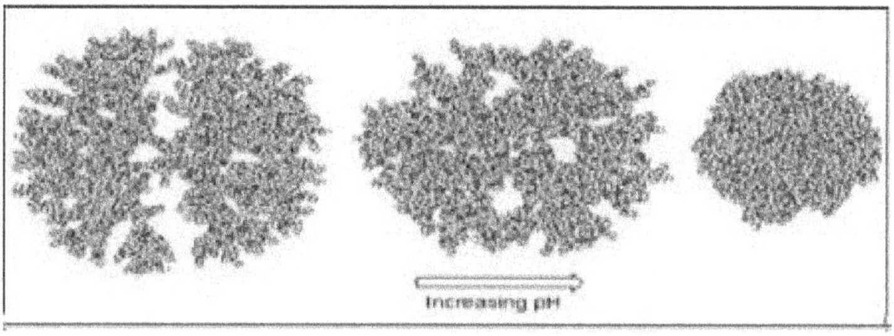

Figure 1.24: Three-dimensional structure of a G6-PAMAM dendrimer, under different pH.

When looking at the pH-dependent conformational changes of **PPI dendrimers having acidic (carboxylic acid) end-groups**, the picture is somewhat different compared to what is observed for their amino-terminated counterparts (Figure 1.25). Small angle neutron scattering (SANS) and NMR measurements of self-diffusion coefficients at different pH values show that at pH 2 the dendrimer core has the most extended conformation due to the electrostatic repulsion between the positively charged protonated tertiary amines, leading to a large radius of the core, whereas the dendrimer reaches its minimum radius at pH 6, where the amount of positively charged amines equals the amount of negatively charged carboxylic groups (isoelectric point) resulting in a "dense core" conformation more subjective to back-folding. Thus, at pH 6 some degree of back-folding occurs as a result of attractive interactions between the negatively charged surface carboxy-groups and the positively charged tertiary amines in the inner shells of the dendrimer. At pH 11 the electrostatic repulsion between the negative charged forces the surface groups apart to give a more extended conformation with a highly expanded surface area (Figure 1.25).

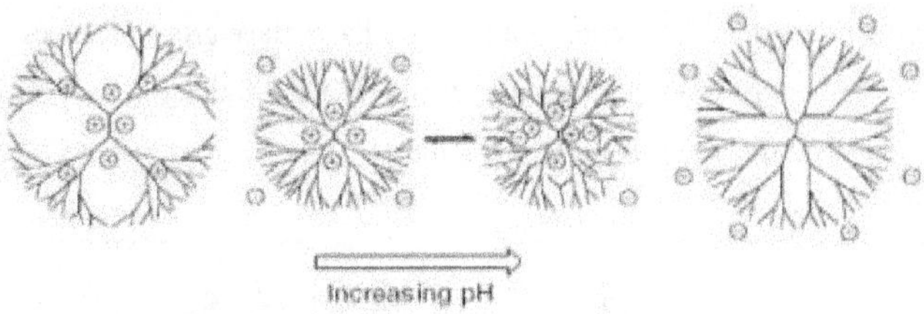

Figure 1.25: Two-dimensional depiction of conformational changes upon different pH of a carboxy-terminated PPI-dendrimer.

Effect of Solvent

The ability of the solvent to solvate the dendrimer structure is a very important parameter when investigating the conformational state of a dendrimer. Dendrimers of all generations generally experience a larger extent of back-folding with decreasing solvent quality, *i.e.* decreasing solvation. However, being more flexible, the low generation dendrimers show the highest tendency towards back-folding as a result of poor solvation compared to the higher generation dendrimers. NMR studies performed on PPI dendrimers conclude that a nonpolar solvent like benzene, poorly solvates the dendrons favouring intramolecular interactions between the dendrimer segments and back-folding. However, a weakly acidic solvent like chloroform can act as a hydrogen donor for the interior amines in a basic dendrimer like PPI, leading to an extended conformation of the dendrimer because of extensive hydrogen bonding between the solvent and the dendrimer amines.[47] Both experimental as well as theoretical studies on amino-terminated PPI and PAMAM dendrimers (polar dendrimers) show the tendency that nonpolar aprotic (poor) solvents induce higher molecular densities in the core region as a result of back-folding, whereas polar (good) solvents solvate the dendrimer arms and induce a higher molecular density on the dendrimer surface. Back-folding of the polar surface groups may expose the more hydrophobic dendrimer parts to the surroundings leading to a decreased surface polarity of the back-folded dendrimer.

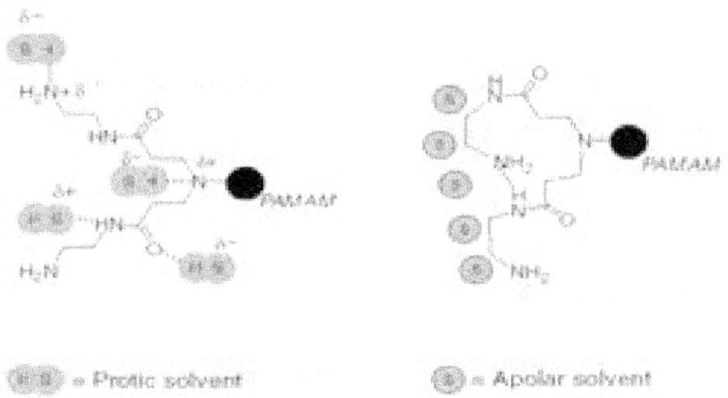

Figure 1.26: Proposed scheme for solvation of a dendrimer under different solvent conditions. (a) Solvation of a polar dendrimer in a protic solvent ("good") leading to extended conformation exposing a polar surface. (b) Solvation of a polar dendrimer in an apolar aprotic solvent ("poor") leading to exposure of an apolar surface consisting of alkyl chains by back-folding.

Effect of Salt

High ionic strength (high concentration of salts) has a strong effect on charged PPI dendrimers and favours a contracted conformation of dendrimers, with a high degree of back-folding somewhat similar to what is observed upon increasing pH or poor salvation. At low salt conditions, the repulsive forces between the charged dendrimer segments results in an extended conformation in order to minimize charge repulsion in the structure (Figure 1.27).

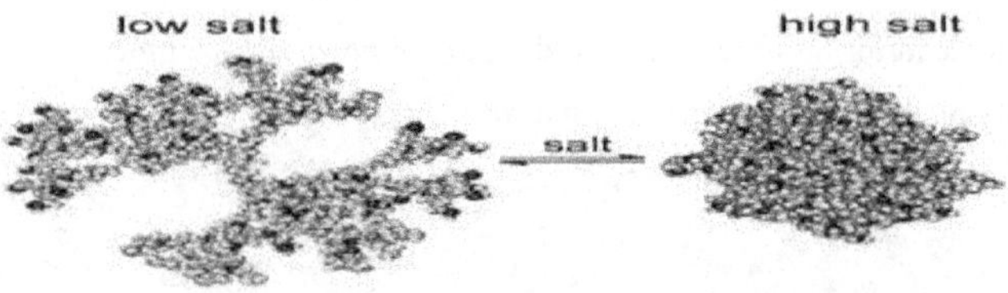

Figure 1.27: The three-dimensional conformational change of a PPI dendrimer upon increasing ionic strength

Effect of Concentration

In dendrimers with flexible structures the conformation is not only affected by small molecules like solvents, salts or protons, but may also be sensitive to larger objects, such as other dendrimers or surfaces which can have a great effect on the molecular density and conformation of the dendrimer. Small angle X-ray scattering (SAXS) experiments performed on PPI dendrimers (G4, G5) in a polar solvent like methanol show that the molecular conformation of dendrimers upon increasing concentration becomes increasingly contracted. This molecular contraction may minimize the repulsive forces between the dendrimer molecules and increase the ability of the dendrimers to exhibit a more tight intermolecular packing.

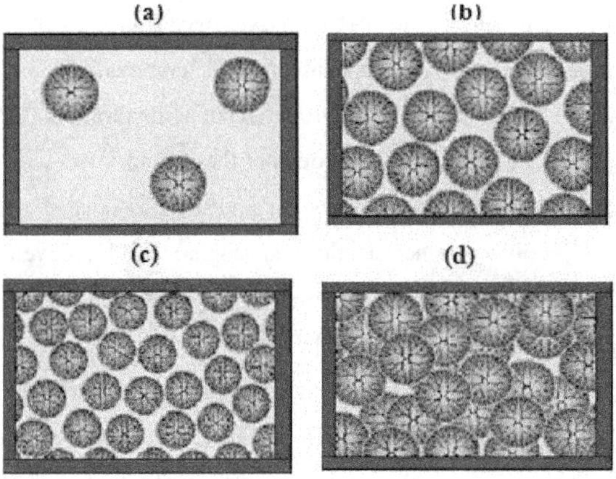

Figure 1.28: Dendrimer at different concentrations (a) Dilute (b) Contact (c) Collapse (d) Interpenetrate

Biological Properties [50-66]

Biological properties of dendrimers are crucial because of the growing interest in using them in biomedical applications. Size is a key determinant of dendrimer cytotoxicity for both PAMAM [50] and PPI dendrimers [51]. Cytotoxicity of PAMAM dendrimers increases with generation for both full generation cationic dendrimers (G2–G4) and the "half-generation" anionic intermediates (G2.5, G3.5) [51, 52, and 53]. The nature and density of charged groups are other factors that determine dendrimer toxicity [52]. Cationic (surface) charges are in general more toxic but details depend on the specific groups involved, that is, for amines it has been proposed that primary amines are relatively more toxic than secondary or tertiary amines. A concentration dependent tendency to cause haemolysis and changes in erythrocyte morphology has been linked to the presence of $-NH_2$ groups [54]. In contrast to PAMAM dendrimers PPI dendrimers with DAB and DAE cores did not show generation dependence for the haemolytic effect [55, 56]. Quaternisation has previously been used as a strategy to reduce toxicity of polymers [57]. The approach also seems to be beneficial for higher generation PPI dendrimers but for complexes the effects of quaternisation are complex and can include changes of complex morphology and physical chemistry, which are difficult to deconvolute [54]. By contrast anionic dendrimers, e.g. those bearing a carboxylate surface are not cytotoxic over a broad concentration range [58, 59]. So despite their broad applicability of commercially available polyamidoamine (PAMAM) dendrimers and Polypropyleneimine dendrimers (PPI), it is generally necessary to modify the surface amine groups of these dendrimers with neutral or anionic moieties to avoid the toxicity and liver accumulation associated with their polycationic surfaces [54, 61]. Polyaryl ether dendrimers (Figure 1.29b), developed by Fréchet and Hawker [62], have been tested for drug delivery applications, but their poor water solubility necessitates the extensive use of solubilizing groups at their periphery [63, 64]. In recent years, much effort has been devoted to the preparation of dendrimers that are designed to be highly biocompatible and water soluble. In addition, some dendrimers have been designed to be biodegradable, and monomer units that are chemical intermediates or products in metabolic pathways have been incorporated. For example, several peptide-based dendrimers, such as those based on polylysine (Figure 1.29c), have been reported, and have been developed as promising vaccine, antiviral and antibacterial candidates after suitable peripheral modifications. Fréchet and co-workers have recently prepared a dendritic analog of the highly biocompatible PEO as a promising backbone for biological applications. Various polyester dendrimers incorporating monomers such as glycerol, succinic acid, phenylalanine and lactic acid (Figure 1.29d) have been prepared by Grinstaff *et al.*, and their potential use in tissue engineering has been demonstrated. Dendritic polymers incorporating glycerol monomers have been developed by Haag [65]. Several other dendrimer families, such as the amides synthesized by Schluter *et al.* and the triazines produced by Simanek *et al.* [66], might also prove to be useful for biological applications.

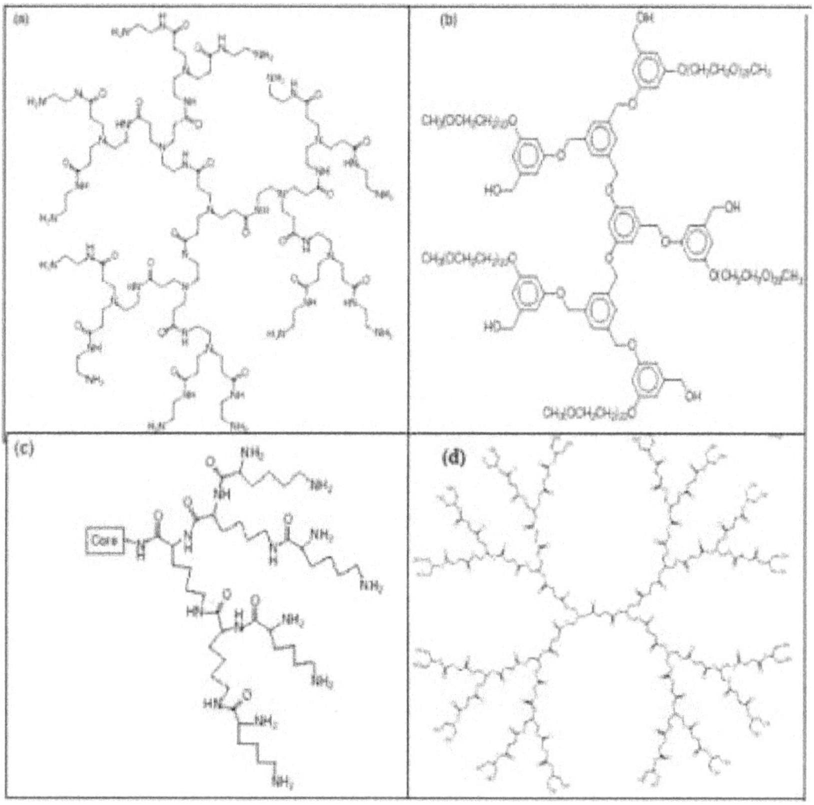

Figure 1.29: Structures of biocompatible dendrimers that have been tested for drug delivery applications. (a) PAMAM dendrimer. (b) Polyaryl ether dendrimer. (c) Polylysine dendron. (d) Polyester dendrimer based on glycerol and succinic acid.

E. Applications [41, 44, 45, 59, 68-71]

Many potential applications of dendrimers are based on their unparalled molecular uniformity, multifunctional surface and presence of internal cavities. These specific properties make dendrimers suitable for a variety of high technology uses and are as follows:

Pharmaceutical Application

Dendrimers Drug Delivery: Targeted and Controlled Release Drug Delivery [41, 45, 59]

Dendrimers have attracted attention as possible drug carriers because of their unique properties namely their well defined three-dimensional structure, the availability of many functional surface groups, their low Polydispersity and their ability to mimic. Drug molecules can be loaded both in the interior of the dendrimers as well as attached to the surface groups. Dendrimers can function as drug carriers either by encapsulating drugs within the dendritic structure, or by inter-acting with drugs at their terminal functional groups via electrostatic or covalent bonds (prodrug).

Delivery of Anticancer Drugs by Dendrimers and Dendritic Polymers [41, 59]

The star polymer gave the most promising results regarding cytotoxicity and systemic circulatory half-life (72 h).In addition to improving drug properties such as solubility and plasma circulation time polymeric carriers can also facilitate the passive targeting of drugs to solid tumors. Combined, these factors lead to the selective accumulation of macromolecules in tumor tissue – a phenomenon termed the 'Enhanced Permeation and Retention' (EPR) effect [51].Therefore, the anticancer drug doxorubicin was covalently bound to this carrier via an acid-labile hydrazone linkage. The cytotoxicity of doxorubicin was significantly reduced (80–98%), and the drug was successfully taken up by several cancer cell lines. The encapsulation behavior of these compounds for the anticancer drugs adriamycin and methotrexate was studied. The highest encapsulation efficiency, with on average 6.5 adriamycin molecules and 26 methotrexate molecules per dendrimer, was found for the G = 4 PAMAM terminated with PEG2000 chains. The anticancer drug 5-fluorouracil encapsulated into G = 4 PAMAM dendrimers with carboxymethyl PEG5000 surface chains revealed reasonable drug loading, and reduced release rate and hemolytic toxicity compared to the non-PEGylated dendrimer(10).In contrast, up to 24 drug molecules were encapsulated into the hyper branched polyol. The drug was successfully transported into lung epithelial carcinoma cells by the dendrimers. Recent studies using Caco-2 cell lines have indicated that low generation PAMAM dendrimers cross cell membranes presumably through a combination of two processes, i.e., paracellular transport and adsorptive endocytosis, while cell efflux systems have a minor effect.

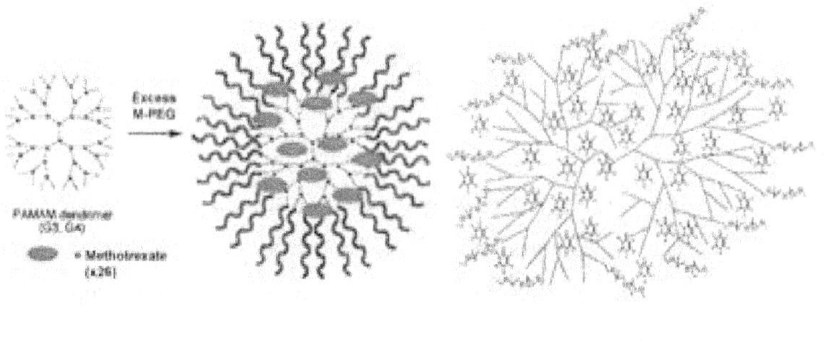

Figure 1.30: The encapsulation of anticancer drugs methotrexate (left) and 5-fluorouracil (right) into PEGylated generation 3 and 4 PAMAM dendrimers [59].

Mechanisms of Drug Delivery [45, 59]

Dendrimers are particularly attractive as they offer a high drug-loading capacity. 2 methods of dendrimer drug delivery are encapsulation of drugs and dendrimer –drug conjugates.

Noncovalent Encapsulation of Drugs / Host –Guest Relation [45, 59]

Encapsulation of drugs uses the satiric bulk of the exterior of the dendrimer or interactions between the dendrimer and drug to trap the drug inside the dendrimer Maciejewski introduced the concept of encapsulating guest molecules into special, egg-shell-like structures [45].Such a system can be used to encapsulate drugs and provide controlled delivery. Initial studies of dendrimers as potential delivery systems focused on their use as unimolecular micelles and 'dendritic boxes' for the noncovalent encapsulation of drug molecules [45].For example, in early studies, DNA was complexed with PAMAM dendrimers for gene delivery applications, and hydrophobic drugs and dye molecules were incorporated into various dendrimer cores. An advantage of using dendritic unimolecular micelles rather than conventional polymeric micelles is that the micellar structure is maintained at all concentrations because the hydrophobic segments are covalently connected. Although the introduction of stabilizing PEO chains on the dendrimer periphery has expanded the scope of den-dritic unimolecular micelles to incorporate anticancer drugs such as 5-fluorouracil methotrexate and doxorubicin and can slow the drug release rates in these systems to some extent [45]. A promising new approach to controlling the release of drugs from the encapsulating micellar compartment involves the use of hybrids of PEO and dendrimers with pH-sensitive hydrophobic acetyl groups on the dendrimer periphery [45].

Covalent Dendrimer–Drug Conjugates [59]

An alternative approach to the development of dendrimers as anticancer drug carriers is to exploit their well-defined multivalency for the covalent attachment of drug molecules to the dendrimer periphery. In dendrimer–drug conjugates, the drug is attached through a covalent bond either directly or via a linker/spacer to the surface groups of a dendrimer. Dendrimers have been conjugated to various biologically active molecules such as drugs, antibodies, sugar moieties and lipids .The drug loading can be tuned by varying the generation number of the dendrimer, and release of the drug can be controlled by incorporating degradable linkages between the drug and dendrimer. Conjugates of PAMAM dendrimers with cisplatin, a potent anticancer drug with non-specific toxicity and poor water solubility .The conjugates show increased solubility, decreased systemic toxicity and selective accumulation in solid tumors. Furthermore, the dendrimer–platinum complex has been found to show increased efficacy relative to cisplatin in the treatment of subcutaneous B16F10 melanoma. By using a careful synthetic strategy with two different chain end functionalities, it is also possible to attach both hydrophobic model drugs and PEO moieties to the dendrimer periphery in a controlled manner. Aliphatic polyester dendrimers based on 2,2-bis(hydroxyethyl)propionic acid are promising dendrimer backbones for the development of anticancer drug conjugates .

Dendrimer as Solubility Enhancers [59, 68]

There are many substances, which have a strong therapeutic activity but due to their lack of solubility in pharmaceutically acceptable solvents have not been used for therapeutic purposes. Water soluble dendrimers are capable of binding and solubilizing small acidic hydrophobic molecules with antifungal or antibacterial properties. Dendrimers having a hydrophobic core and a hydrophilic surface layer have been termed unimolecular micelles. Unlike traditional micelles, dendrimers do not have a critical micelle concentration. This characteristic offers the opportunity to soluble poorly soluble drugs by encapsulating them within the dendritic structure at all concentrations of dendrimer. A hydrophilic–hydrophobic core-shell dendrimer with PAMAM interior and long alkane chain exterior was shown to bind 5-flurouracil, a water-soluble anti-tumor drug [59].After phospholipid coating of the dendrimer–fatty- acid macromolecule, oral bioavailability in rats of 5-flurouracil was nearly twice the level of free 5-flurouracil . Dendrimer-based carriers could offer the opportunity to enhance the oral bioavailability of problematic drugs. Propranolol, conjugated to surface-modified G3 PAMAM dendrimer, the solubility of propranolol increased by over two orders of magnitude. Thus, dendrimer nanocarriers offer the potential to enhance the bioavailability of drugs that are poorly soluble and/or substrates for efflux transporters [68].

Cellular Delivery Using Dendrimer Carriers [68]

Kannan et al. studied the dynamics of cellular entry into A549 human lung epithelial carcinoma cells of a range of PAMAM dendrimers (G4-NH_2, G3-NH_2, G4-OH, PEGylated G3 [G3-PEG]) and a hyper branched polymer (polyol). G4-$NH_2$and G4-OH entered cells more rapidly than did G3-NH_2, polyol or G3-PEG. It was suggested that the rapid entry of G4-NH_2 might be a result of the cationic nature of the amine surface groups, which may interact electrostatically with negatively charged epithelial cells and enter via fluid phase pinocytosis. The lower rate of cellular entry of G3-NH_2com-pared with G4-NH_2may is a result of fewer surface charges on the G3-NH_2dendrimer[68].Because polyol and G3-PEG do not have cationic surface groups, their cellular entry may result from non-specific adsorption to the cell membrane and subsequent endocytosis. Dendrimer–ibuprofen complexes entered the cells rapidly compared with pure drug (1 hr versus>3 hr), suggesting that dendrimers can efficiently carry the complexed drug inside cells. PAMAM dendrimers were surface-engineered with lauryl chains to reduce toxicity and enhance cellular uptake.

Dendrimers as Nano-Drugs [41]

Poly(lysine) dendrimers modified with sulfonated naphthyl groups have been found to be useful as antiviral drugs against the herpes simplex virus can potentially prevent/reduce transmission of HIV and other sexually transmitted diseases (STDs) [41].In earlier studies, it was found that PAMAM dendrimers covalently modified with naphthyl sulfonate residues on the surface, also exhibited antiviral activity against HIV. This dendrimer-based nano-drug inhibited early stage virus/cell adsorption and later stage viral replication by interfering with reverse transcriptase and/or integrase enzyme activities. PPI dendrimers with tertiary alkyl ammonium groups attached to the surface have been shown to be potent antibacterial biocides against Gram positive and Gram negative bacteria. Poly (lysine) dendrimers with mannosyl surface groups are effective inhibitors of the adhesion of E. coli to horse blood cells in a haemagglutination assay, making these structures promising antibacterial agents. Chitosan–dendrimer hybrids have been found to be useful as antibacterial agents, carriers in drug delivery systems, and in other biomedical applications.

Dendrimers in Photodynamic Therapy (PDT)[41, 59]

The photosensitizer 5-aminolevulinic acid has been attached to the surface of dendrimers and studied as an agent for PDT of tumorigenic keratinocytes .Photos sensitive dyes have been incorporated into dendrimers and utilized in PDT devices [41]. This cancer treatment involves the administration of a light- activated photosensitizing drug that selectively concentrates in diseased tissue. The possibility of improving the properties of dendrimers through appropriate unfunctionalization of their periphery makes dendrimers promising carriers for photosensitizers. ALA is a natural precursor of the photosensitizer protoporphyrin IX (PIX), and its administration is known to increase cellular concentrations of PIX [59].

Dendrimers in Gene Transfection [41, 44]

Dendrimers can act as **vectors, in gene therapy**. PAMAM dendrimers have been tested as genetic material carriers. Numerous reports have been published describing the use of amino-terminated PAMAM or PPI dendrimers as non-viral gene transfer agents, enhancing the transfection of DNA by endocytosis and, ultimately, into the cell nucleus [41]. A transfection reagent called SuperFectTM consisting of activated dendrimers is commercially available. Activated dendrimers can carry a larger amount of genetic material than viruses. SuperFect–DNA complexes are characterized by high stability and provide more efficient transport of DNA into the nucleus than liposomes. The high transfection efficiency of dendrimers may not only be due to their well-defined shape but may also be caused by the low pK of the amines (3.9 and 6.9). The low p*K* permit the dendrimer to buffer the pH change in the endosomal Compartment [44]. PAMAM dendrimers functionalized with cyclodextrin showed luciferase gene expression about 100 times higher than for unfunctionalized PAMAM or for non-covalent mixtures of PAMAM and cyclodextrin. It should be noted that dendrimers of high structural flexibility and partially degraded high-generation dendrimers (i.e., hyper branched architectures) appear to be better suited for certain gene delivery operations than intact high-generation symmetrical Dendrimers [41] .

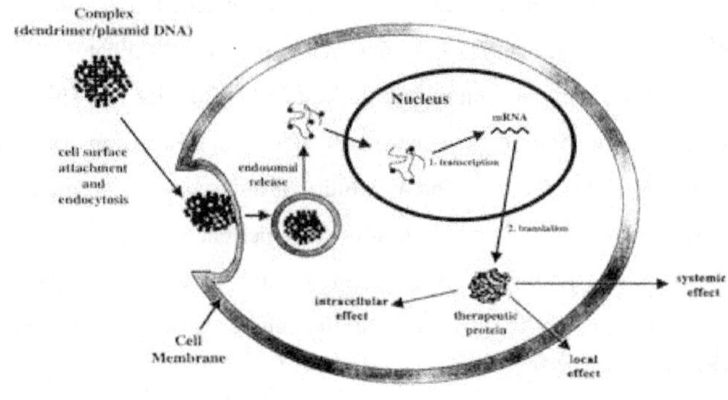

Figure 1.31: Dendrimer involved in gene transfection

In nutshell dendrimers holds a promising future in various pharmaceutical applications and diagnostic field in the coming years as they possess unique properties, such as high degree of branching, multivalency, globular architecture and well-defined molecular weight, thereby offering new scaffolds for drug delivery. An increasingly large number of drugs being developed today facing problems of short half-life, poor solubility, bioavailability and permeability. Dendrimers can work as a useful tool for optimizing drug delivery of such problematic drugs. Also the problem of biocompatibility and toxicity can be overcome by careful surface engineering. Recent successes in simplifying and optimizing the synthesis of dendrimers provide a large variety of structures with reduced cost of their production. Also as research progresses, newer applications of dendrimers will emerge and the future should witness an increasing numbers of commercialized dendrimer based drug delivery systems.

1.4 ORIGIN AND OBJECTIVES OF RESEARCH WORK

Half life is the period of time required for the concentration or amount of drug in the body to be reduced by one-half. We usually consider the half life of a drug in relation to the amount of the drug in plasma.

Therapeutically active agents, however, often suffer from number of shortcomings which limit and complicate their use. A particular problem is short half life of drugs, after administration to the patient; a drug may be so rapidly cleared from the body by metabolic or other pathways or otherwise biologically inactivated so that only a relatively small percentage of the drug administered actually has a therapeutic effect for example many over the counter pain relievers like ibuprofen and medications that are used as tranquilizers like benzodiazepines have notoriously short half lives.

To compensate for this problem, it is common practice to increase the dose of the drug and or to prolong its period of administration and or to shorten the interval between doses so that the therapeutically effective concentration of the drug in the patient is maintained for a period sufficient to achieve the desired result.

These procedures are useful but have their own limitations. Increasing the dose may be limited, for example, in the case of intramuscular administration, by the bolus which can be tolerated. Many drugs have toxic side effects which may limit the dose duration or interval which can be safely used. In some cases, promising drugs cannot be used because side reactions are so severe that an effective therapeutic dose cannot be safely administered. The need to administer multiple small doses of a drug or to use continuous infusion techniques increases the cost of treatment and the burden on hospital personnel, and of course, adds to the patient's discomfort. Accordingly there **exists a need** for means by which the therapeutically active concentration of a drug after administration is maintained for a longer time.

Objectives

The main objectives of the study are as under:

1. To reduce the dosing frequency.
2. To improve patient convenience and compliance.
3. To minimize dose by maximum utilization of drug for therapeutic effect via reduction of unavoidable wastage of drug through fast elimination.
4. To extend the duration of action of drug.
5. To reduce health care cost and improves safe use of drug.

In literature survey it is found that there are mainly two approaches to increase serum half-life ($t_{1/2}$) of a drug, which are as following-

1.) By decreasing drug metabolism (pharmaceutical, pharmacological and chemical approaches described in section 1.2)

A simple example of this type of modification is Chlorpropamide which is derived from Tolbutamide having short half life used as oral hypoglycemic.

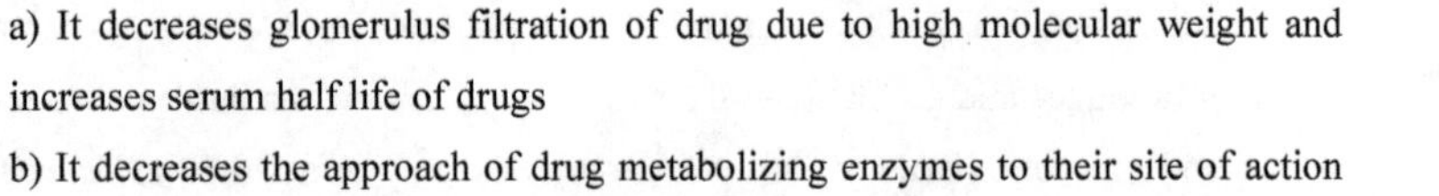

($t_{1/2}$ = 4.5 to 6.5 hrs) ($t_{1/2}$ = 36 hrs)

Tolbutamide Chlorpropamide

2.) By increasing molecular weight of drug by polymer binding to drug-

a) It decreases glomerulus filtration of drug due to high molecular weight and increases serum half life of drugs

b) It decreases the approach of drug metabolizing enzymes to their site of action on the drug molecule due to steric hindrance of polymer bound drug thus half life of drug increases.

1.5 PLAN OF WORK

The research is planned and would be executed on the following lines:

- Selection & Authentification of target drugs for Derivatization
- Selection of reaction and kind of derivatives to be prepared
- Structural Derivatization / modification in the selected drugs reducing its elimination through the body to increase its half life.
- Characterization of the derivatized drugs.
- *In-vitro* studies of derivatized drugs.
- *In-vivo* studies of derivatized drugs.

REFERENCES

1. L.Z. Benet, J.R. Mitchell, and L.B. Sheiner in A.G. Gilman, T.W. Rall, A.S. Nies, and P. Taylor, Eds., Goodman and Gilman's The Pharmacological Basis of Therapeutics, Pergamon Press, Elmsford, NY, 1990, 3-32.

2. L.Z. Benet and R.L. Williams in A.G. Gilman, T.W. Rall, A.S. Nies, and P. Taylor, Eds., Goodman and Gilman's The Pharmacological Basis of Therapeutics, Pergamon Press, Elmsford, NY, 1990, 1650-1735.

3. K.S. Pang and M.Rowland, Hepatic clearance of drugs. J. Pharmacokinet. Biopharm., 5, 625-653 (1977).

4. H. Boxenbaum, Interspecies variation in liver weight, hepatic blood flow, and antipyrine intrinsic clearance: extrapolation of data to benzodiazepine and phenytoin J. Pharmacokinet. Biopharm. 8, 165-170 (1980).

5. J. Mordenti, S.A. Chen, J.A. Moore, B.L. Ferraiolo, and J.D. Green, Interspecies scaling of clearance and volume of distribution data for five therapeutic proteins. Pharm. Res., 8, 1351-1359 (1991).

6. M.F. Hebert, J.P. Roberts, T.Prueksaritanont, and L.Z. Benet, Bioavailability of cyclosporine with concomitant rifampin administration is markedly less than predicted by hepatic enzyme induction. Clin. Pharmacol, Ther., 52, 453-457 (1992).

7. R.J. Wills, S.Dennis, H.E. Spiegel, D.M. Gibson, and P.I. Nadler, Interferon kinetics and adverse reactions after intravenous, intramuscular, and subcutaneous injection. Clin. Pharmacol. Ther., 35, 722-727 (1984).

8. L.Z. Benet and R.L. Galeazzi, Noncompartmental determination of the volume of distribution steady-state. J. Pharm. Sci., 68, 1071-1074 (1979).

9. U. Klotz, G.R. Avant, A.Hoyumpa, S. Schenker, and G.R. Wilkinson, The effects of age and liver disease on the disposition and elimination of diazepam in adult man. J. Clin. Invest., 55, 347-359, (1975).

10. R.L. Williams, T.F. Blaschke, P.J. Meffin, K.L.Melmon, and M. Rowland, Nanomedicine and personalized medicine toward the application of pharmacotyping Clin. Pharmacol. Ther., 21, 301-409 (1977).

11. B.L. Ferraiolo and L.Z. Benet in R.T. Borchard, A.J.Repta, and V.J. Stella, Eds., Directed Drug Delivery: The Multi-disciplinary problem, Humana Press, Clifton, NJ, 1985, 13-33.

12. C.A. Gloff and L.Z. Benet, Pharmacokinetics and protein therapeutics. Adv. Drug Deliv. Rev., 4, 359-386 (1990)

13. Shargel L., Mutnick A.H., Souney P.F., Swanson L.N.; Comprehensive Pharmacy Review; Published by Wolterskluwer (India) Pvt. Ltd., New Delhi, sixth edition, 404-405.

14. Patrick. Graham. L, An introduction to medicinal chemistry. Oxford university press, New York, Fourth edition, 245-249.

15. Ringsdorf, H. Synthetic Polymeric Drugs, In Polymeric Delivery Systems; Kostelnik, R.J., Ed.; Gordon and Breach Science Publishers, Inc.: New York, 1978; 197- 225.

16. Ringsdorf, H. Structure and properties of pharmacologically active polymers.J. Polym. Sci., Symp. 51, 135-153 (1975)

17. Christie, R.J.; Grainger, D.W. Design strategies to improve soluble macromolecular delivery constructs. Adv. Drug Deliv. Rev. 55, 421- 437 (2003).

18. Abuchowski, A.; Van Es, T.; Palzuk, N.C.; Davis, F.F. Effect of covalent attachment of polyethylene glycol on immunogenicity and circulating life of bovine liver catalase. J. Biol. Chem. 2, 3578-3581 (1977).

19. Hooftman, G.; Herman, S.; Schacht, E. Review: poly (ethylene glycol)s with reactive endgroups. II. Practical consideration for the preparation of protein-PEG conjugates. J. Bioact. Compat. Polymers 11, 135-159 (1996).

20. Zalipsky, S. Chemistry of polyethylene glycol conjugates with biologically active molecules. Adv.Drug Delivery Rev. 16, 157-182 (1995).

21. Fuke, I.; Toshio, H.; Tabata, Y.; Ikada, Y. Synthesis of PEG derivatives with different branching and their use for protein modification. J. Control. Rel. 30, 27-34 (1994).

22. Roberts, M.J., Bentley, M.D., Harris, J.M. Chemistry for peptide and protein PEGylation.. Adv. Drug Deliv. Rev. 54, 459-476 (2002).

23. Chapman, A.P. *et al.* Therapeutic antibody fragments with prolonged in vivo half-lives. Nature Biotechnol. 17, 780-783 (1999).

24. Sato, H. Enzymatic procedure for site-specific pegylation of proteins. Adv. Drug Deliv. Rev. 54, 487-504 (2002).

25. Vellard, M. The enzyme as drug: application of enzymes as pharmaceuticals. Curr. Opin. Biotechnol. 14, 1-7 (2003).

26. Reddy K. R., Modi, M. W. & Pedder, S. Use of peginterferon a-2a (40 KD) (Pegasys) for the treatment of hepatitis C. Adv. Drug Deli. Rev. 54, 571-586 (2002).

27. Schiavon, O.; Pasut, G.; Moro, S.; Orsolini, P.; Guiotto, A.; Veronese, F.M. PEG-Ara-C conjugates for controlled release. Eur. J. Med. Chem. 39, 123-133 (2004).

28. Denis, L. *et al.* Proc. Am. Soc. Clin. Oncol. 19, 700 (2000);
Greenwald, R.B. *et al.* Adv. Drug. Deliv. Rev. 55, 217-250 (2003).

29. Duncan, R. The Dawning Era of Polymer Therapeutics. Nat. Rev. Drug. Discov. 2, 347-360 (2003)

30. Greenwald, R.B.; Choe, Y.H.; McGuire, J.; Conover, C.D. Effective drug delivery by PEGylated drug conjugates. Adv. Drug Deliv. Rev. 55, 217-250 (2003).

31. Greenwald, R.B. PEG drugs: an overview. J. Control. Rel. 74, 159-171 (2001).

32. Buhleier E, Wehner W and Vogtle F, "Cascade and Nonskid-chain-like Synthesis of Molecular Cavity Topologies", Synthesis, 2, 155-158, (1978).

33. Tomalia D.A, Baker H, Dewald J, Hall M, Kallos G, Martin S, Roeck J, Ryder J and Smith P, "A New Class of Polymers: Starburst-Dendritic Macromolecules", Polym. J., 17, 117-132, (1985).

34. Newkome G.R, Yao Z.Q, Baker G.R and Gupta V.K, "Cascade molecules: A new approach to micelles, A", J. Org. Chem., 50, 2003–2006, (1985).

35. Pushkar S, Philip A, Pathak K and Pathak D, "Dendrimers: Nanotechnology Derived Novel Polymers in Drug Delivery", Indian J. Pharm. Educ. Res., 40, 153-158, (2006).

36. Sakthivel T and Florence A.T, "Adsorption of Amphipathic Dendrons on Polystyrene Nanoparticles", Int. J. Pharm., 254, 23-26, (2003).

37. Yiyun C, Zhenhua X, Minglu M and Tonguen X, "Dendrimers as Drug Carriers: Applications in Different Routes of Drug", J.Pharma.Sci, 97, 123-143, (2008).

38. Hawker C and Fréchet J.M.J, "A new convergent approach to monodisperse dendritic molecule" J. Chem. Soc. Chem. Commun., 15, 1010-1012, (1990).

39. Hawker C, Wooley K.L and Fréchet J.M.J, Fullerene-bound Dendrimers: Soluble, Isolated Carbon Clusters. J.Chem. Soc. Perkin. Trans., 1, 1287-1289, (1993).

40. Frechet J.M.J and Tomalia D.A, "Introduction to the Dendritic state", Dendrimers and other Dendritic Polymers, John Wiley & Sons Ltd, 24-23, (2001).

41. Sonke S and Tomalia D.A, "Dendrimers in biomedical applications reflections on the Field", Advanced Drug Delivery Reviews, 57, 2106 – 2129, (2005).

42. Christine D, Ijeoma F.U and Andreas G.S, "Dendrimers in gene delivery", Advanced Drug Delivery Reviews, 57, 2177– 2202, (2005).

43. Freeman A.W and Frechet J.M.J, "Developments in the Accelerated Convergent Synthesis of Dendrimers", Dendrimers and other Dendritic Polymers Edited by Jean M. J. Fre´chet and Donald A. Tomalia, 91-101.

44. Barbara K. and Maria B., "*Review* Dendrimers: properties and applications", Acta Biochimica Polonica, 48, 199–208 (2001).

45. R.P.Patel et al. "Dendrimers: A new innovation in drug delivery", Pharma Bio World, 42-52 (2007).

46. Boris D, Rubinstein M, "A self-consistent mean field model of a starburst dendrimer: dense core vs. dense shell", Macromolecules, 29, 7251– 7260 (1996).

47. Chai M, Niu Y., Youngs W.J and Rinaldi P.L, "Structure and conformation of DAB dendrimers in solution via multidimensional NMR techniques", J. Am. Chem. Soc., 123, 4670– 4678 (2001).

48. Gupta U, Agashe H and Jain N.K, "Polypropylene imine dendrimer mediated solubility enhancement: effect of pH and functional groups of hydrophobes", J. Pharm. Sci., 10, 358-67 (2007).

49. Wang D.J and Imae T, "fluorescence emission from Dendrimer & its pH dependence", J. Am. Chem. Soc., 126, 13204-13205 (2004).

50. Zinselmeyer B.H, Mackay S.P, Schatzlein A.G and Uchegbu I.F, "The lower-generation polypropylenimine dendrimers are effective gene-transfer agents", Pharm. Res., 19, 960– 967 (2002).

51. Jevprasesphant R, Penny J, Jalal R, Attwood D, McKeown N.B and D'Emanuele A., "The influence of surface modification on the cytotoxicity of PAMAM dendrimers", Int. J. Pharm., 252, 263– 266 (2003).

52. Jevprasesphant R, Penny J, Jalal R, Attwood D, McKeown N.B and D'Emanuele A., "Engineering of dendrimer surfaces to enhance transepithelial transport and reduce cytotoxicity", Pharm. Res. 20, 1543– 1550 (2003).

53. Satija J, Gupta U and Jain N.K "Pharmaceutical and biomedical potential of surface engineered dendrimers" Crit Rev Ther Drug Carrier Syst., 24, 257-306 (2007).

54. Malik N, Wiwattanapatapee R, Klopsch R, Lorenz K, Frey H, Weener J.W, Meijer E.W, Paulus W and Duncan R, "Dendrimers: relationship between structure and

biocompatibility in vitro, and preliminary studies on the biodistribution of I-125-labelled polyamidoamine dendrimers in vivo", J.Control. Release, 65, 133– 148 (2000).

55. Uchegbu I.F, Sadiq L, Pardakhty A, El-Hammadi M, Gray A.I, Tetley L, Wang W, Zinselmeyer B.H and Schatzlein A.G, "Gene transfer with three amphiphilic glycol chitosans —the degree of polymerization is the main controller of transfection efficiency", J. Drug Target., 12, 527–539 (2004).

56. Brownlie A, Uchegbu I.F and Schatzlein A.G, "PEI-based vesicle-polymer hybrid gene delivery system with improved biocompatibility", Int. J. Pharm., 274, 41– 52 (2004).

57. Schatzlein A.G, Zinselmeyer B.H, Elouzi A, Dufes C, Chim Y.T, Roberts C.J, Davies M.C, Munro A, Gray A.I and Uchegbu I.F, "Preferential liver gene expression with polypropylenimine dendrimers", J. Control. Release, 101, 247– 258 (2005).

58. Chen H.T, Neerman M.F, Parrish A.R and Simanek E.E, "Cytotoxicity, haemolysis, and acute in vivo toxicity of dendrimers based on melamine, candidate vehicles for drug delivery", J. Am. Chem. Soc., 126, 10044– 10048 (2004).

59. Gillies E.R. and Fréchet J.M.J, "Dendrimers and dendritic polymers in drug delivery" Drug Discovery Today, 10, 35-43 (2005).

60. Esfand, R. and Tomalia, D.A. "Polyamidoamine (PAMAM) dendrimers: from biomimicry to drug delivery and biomedical applications". Drug Discov. Today, 6, 427–436 (2001).

61. Jevpraesesphant, R. *et al.*, "The influence of surface modification on the cytotoxicity of PAMAM dendrimers", Int.J. Pharm., 252, 263–266 (2003).

62. Hawker, C.J. and Fréchet, J.M.J. "Preparation of polymers with controlled molecular architecture. A new convergent approach to dendritic macromolecules". J. Am.Chem. Soc., 112, 7638–7647 (1990).

63. Liu, M. *et al.* "Water-soluble unimolecular micelles: their potential as drug delivery agents". J. Control. Release, 65, 121–131 (2000).

64. Liu, M. *et al.* "Water-soluble dendrimer–polyethylene glycol starlike conjugates as potential drug carriers". J. Polym. Sci, 37, 3492–3503 (1999).

65. Haag, R. *et al.* "An approach to glycerol dendrimers and pseudo-dendritic polyglycerols". J. Am. Chem. Soc., 122, 2954–2955 (2000).

66. Neerman M.F *et al.* "*In vitro* and *in vivo* evaluation of a melamine dendrimer as a vehicle for drug delivery". Int. J. Pharm., 281, 129–132 (2004).

67. Caminade A.M, Laurent R. and Majoral J.P, "Characterization of dendrimers", Advanced Drug Delivery Reviews, 57, 2130-2146 (2005).

68. Mohammad N and Antony D, "Crossing cellular barriers using dendrimer nanotechnologies", Current Opinion in Pharmacology, 6, 522–527 (2006).

69. Lee S.C "Dendrimers in Nanobiological Devices", Dendrimers and other Dendritic Polymers Edited by Fre´chet J.M.J and Tomalia D.A., 547-554.

70. Kleij A.W, Ford A, JastrzebskI H and Vankoten G, "Dendritic Polymer Applications: Catalysts", Edited by Fre´chet J.M.J and Tomalia D.A., 485-507.

71. Kofoed J and Reymond J, "Dendrimers as artificial enzymes", Current Opinion in Chemical Biology, 9, 656–664 (2005).

Any success story always begins with the careful selection, proper identification of quality and purity of the materials required in the project. Research envisages the derivatization of drugs for the enhancement of half-life. Therefore, it is necessary to have a look for eligible candidates in selection of the drugs.

For the selection of drugs main criteria was that drug should have short biological half-life, its frequency of administration is higher and drug should have functional group that can be bonded with polyethylene glycols, thus it shall have groups like –COOH, -SO_3H etc. So that further derivatization can take place.

Based on the above considerations the following drugs were selected for derivatization and half-life enhancement.

- **Cloxacillin**
- **Cephalexin**
- **Ciprofloxacin**

Only the selection of drugs, for derivatization, is not sufficient unless the complete characterization and proper methods of quantitative estimations are also selected. For such selection complete awareness about the profiles of drugs is required. Their characteristics reported in the literature were collected and described as the profile of individual drug; however the literature available on these drugs is very bulky. Therefore, only a part of it was selected on the basis of relevance. The drugs were tested for quality on the basis of their pharmacopoeial monographs. Hence, the characterization is described along with the profile. The analytical methods are required for the quantitative analyses of drugs in plasma. The methods selected for such purpose are described along with the profile of individual drugs.

2.1 CLOXACILLIN SODIUM

2.1.1 Drug Profile

2.1.1.1 Description[1]

Name, Formula, Molecular Weight

Sodium Cloxacillin is found in Chemical Abstracts under 4-Thia-1-azabicyclo [3.2.0] heptane-2-carboxylic acid, 6-[[[3-(2-chlorophenyl)-5-methyl-4-isoxazoyl] carbonyl] amino] -3, 3-dimethyl-7-oxo-monosodium salt. It is more commonly known as 3-o-chlorophenyl-5-methyl-4-isoxazolyl penicillin sodium salt.

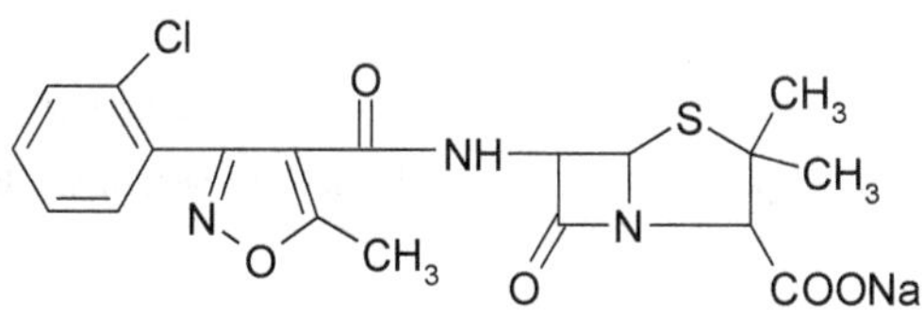

$C_{19}H_{17}ClN_3NaO_5S$ Molecular Weight = 457.89

Appearance

Sodium cloxacillin is a white, odorless, crystalline powder.

2.1.1.2 Physical Properties[1]

Infrared Spectrum

Infrared absorption frequencies were reported for oil suspension of cloxacillin and other penicillins by E. A. Rudzit et. al. A spectrogram of Bristol Laboratories Primary Reference Standard recorded as a potassium bromide disk using a Beckman Model IR9 Spectrometer is shown in Fig. 2.1. Characteristic absorption frequencies (cm^{-1}) are as follows:

a. H_2O	3519
b. N-H stretching band	3370
c. beta-lactam carbonyl	1770
d. secondary amide carbonyl	1669
e. aromatic ring	1619
f. carboxylate carbonyl	1604

Within the carbonyl stretching region, the beta-lactam frequency is most characteristic of penicillins. Opening of the beta-lactam can be indicated by changes in this part of the spectrum.

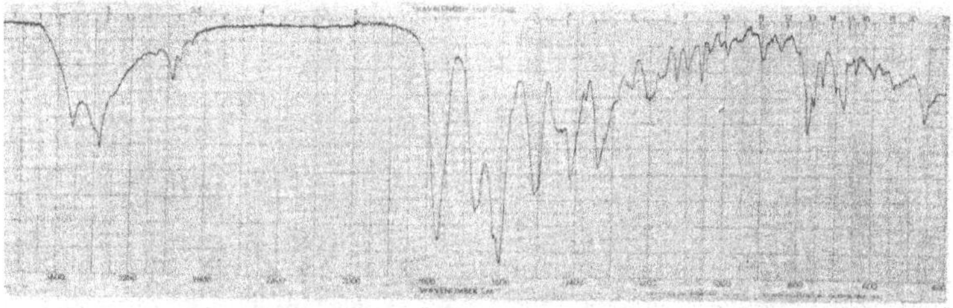

Figure 2.1 Infrared absorption spectrum of sodium cloxacillin monohydrate

Nuclear Magnetic Resonance Spectra

Proton nuclear magnetic resonance spectra for a number of penicillins were reported by Pek and coworkers and the chemical shifts useful for identification were tabulated. An nmr spectrogram of Bristol Laboratories Primary Reference Standard sodium cloxacillin monohydrate as obtained on a Varian HA-100 spectrometer is shown in Figure 2.2. Protons resonance lines were measured in D_2O solution with Deuterated sodium trimethylsilyl propionate as the internal reference. Structural assignments are as follows:

Assignment	**Chemical Shift, (Coupling Constant, Hz)**
Aromatic	7.50 m
6-H	5.62 d (J=4.0)
5-H	5.46 d (J=4.0)
3-H	4.81 s
5-CH_3 (isoxazole)	2.63 s
2-β-CH_3	1.43 s
2-α-CH_3	1.39 s

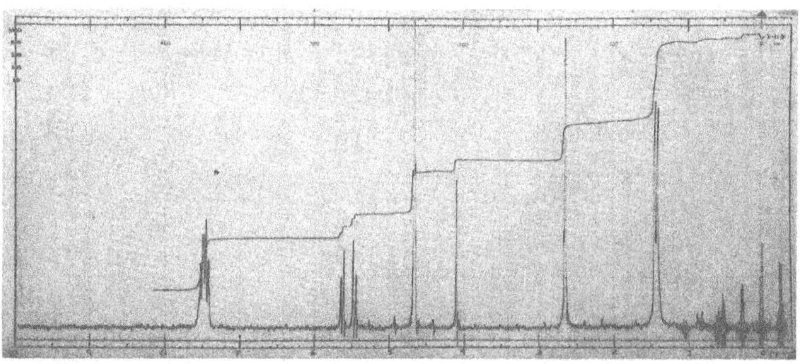

NMR spectrum of sodium cloxacillin monohydrate

Figure 2.2 NMR spectrum of sodium cloxacillin monohydrate

Crystal Properties

Sodium cloxacillin is a microcrystalline powder exhibiting birefringence and extinction positions under a light polarizing microscope.

Melting Range

Sodium cloxacillin melts with decomposition at 170°C. Cloxacillin free acid melts with decomposition at 126-127°C.

Solubility

Sodium cloxacillin is very soluble in cold water. The ratio of sodium cloxacillin concentration in chloroform versus pH 6 buffer solution was determined to be 0.118. The solubility of penicillin salts in nonpolar solvents is significantly increased by the presence of a small amount of water, even water of hydration, also soluble in methanol, ethanol, pyridine and ethylene glycol.

Ionization Constant pKa

Budgaard and Ilver reported an apparent pKa of 2.68 ± 0.05 at 35°C., determined by measuring the pH of a partially neutralized 0.0025 M solution of sodium cloxacillin. Rapson and Bird obtained replicate apparent pK values of 2.73 ± 0.04 and 2.70 ± 0.03 at 25°C. by titrating 0.0025 M sodium cloxacillin solutions.

Optical Rotation

Cloxacillin has 3 asymmetric carbon atoms and is strongly dextrorotatory. Specific rotation values in the literature are shown below:

Cloxacillin	$[\alpha]_D$	Temp.	Conc. And Solvent
Sodium salt	+ 163°	20°C	1% in water
Free acid	+122°	20°C	1% in acetone

2.1.1.3 Methods of Analyses[1]

Identification Tests

Sodium cloxacillin is identified by the infrared absorption spectrum and by the penicillin characteristic purple colour formed upon treatment with chromotropic acid in sulfuric acid at 150°C.

Quantitative Methods:

Volumetric Methods

Iodine is not consumed by penicillins but is consumed by the hydrolysis products. The difference in iodine consumption before and after alkaline hydrolysis is used as a standard method of determining cloxacillin content.

Hydrolysis with a measured excess of alkali generates an additional carboxyl group in the penicilloic acid. Back titration of the excess alkali with hydrochloric acid is used for determination of cloxacillin content.

Colorimetric Methods

Cloxacillin has been determined by measurement of the side chain absorbance at 275 nm. Penicillin have been determined by measurement of the absorption maximum near 340 nm produced by acid degradation to the corresponding penicillenic acids. Formation of the penicillanic acid is catalyzed by copper and other metals and by imidazole.

Penicillins have long been determined by reaction with hydroxylamine. The hydroxamic acids generated produce a red-colored chelate with iron (III). Details of the procedure are available in the Federal Register. Automated versions of the method have also been used.

Polarography

Penicillins in serum were determined by polarographic techniques. The analysis required about two hours. Cloxacillin was determined at levels of 5 μg/ml in sulfuric acid solution.

Gas Chromatography

Organic acid side chains produced by vigorous alkaline hydrolysis of penicillins were converted to methyl esters for gas chromatographic separation on a 3.5% SE-30 column. Intact penicillins were gas chromatographed as the corresponding methyl esters on a 2% fluoro-silicone phase by Martin and coworkers. Separation of the trimethylsilyl esters of several penicillins on a 2% OV-17 column was reported by Hishta, et. al. Cloxacillin was separated from several other penicillins and quantitation was indicated by reproducibility of response factors on reference samples.

Infrared Spectroscopy

The infrared absorption due to the beta-lactam has been used to quantitate penicillins after extraction into a suitable solvent. The cloxacillin beta-lactam band near 1760 cm^{-1} was used to measure cloxacillin inactivation by beta-lactamase as differentiated from amidase. For this work solutions were lyophilized in the presence of potassium bromide and infrared absorption measurements were made from the solid disks.

Optical Rotation

The change in optical rotation upon treatment with penicillinases has been used to quantitate penicillins. Penicillins which are more susceptible to penicillinases can be determined in the presence of resistant penicillins. Ampicillin and cloxacillin were determined in combination.

Biological Methods

The cylinder plate agar diffusion method is the official microbiological method of determination. Staph aureus (ATCC 6538P) is the organism of choice. Cloxacillin has been microbiologically determined in the presence of Ampicillin using agar impregnated with penicillinase to destroy the Ampicillin activity or after ion exchange separation on a column of iRA-402. Cloxacillin is routinely measured by the turbidimetric method using Staph aureus FDA-209P (ATCC 6538P) or Staph aureus BL-A9596.

A microbiological paper disk procedure has been described for measuring cloxacillin and other antibiotics in as little as 10μl of plasma. Hooke and Ball used an agar plate method and Sarcina lutea NCIB 8553 to measure cloxacillin at levels below 10 μg/ml in milk.

In a test to detect trace levels in milk, penicillin inhibits growth of Streptococcus thermophilus B.C., which otherwise causes the dye 2, 3, 5-triphenyltetrazolium chloride, to turn from colorless to red. Other antibiotics interfere.

Automated Methods

Several chemical methods for penicillin determination have been automated, including the hydroxylamine methods, the iodometric method, the penicillenic acid method, and a colorimetric method based on enzyme deacylation to 6-amino penicillanic acid and detection with p-dimethylamino benzaldehyde. Cloxacillin, specifically, is mentioned in the hydroxylamine and penicillanic acid automated procedures.

Thin-layer Chromatography

Reviews on chromatography and analysis of antibiotics are available. Cloxacillin has been chromatographed on paper, kieselguhr G, cellulose, commercial silica gel plates and silica gel G predeveloped with silicone (5% DC 200 in ether).

Cloxacillin has been separated from other penicillins, and from impurities, from cephalosporins, from other antibiotics, and from constituents of body fluids.
Chromatography has been used to study solvent partitioning and structure activity relationships.
Visualization spray reagents used include iodine-azide solution followed by aqueous starch to give white spots on blue purple; 10% acetic acid in acetone followed by starch-iodine to give white spots on blue; ammoniated copper sulfate; 0.5% bromine solution; 0.25% fluorescein; ferric chloride and potassium ferricyanide with sulfuric acid to give blue spots on green; alkaline potassium permanganate and heat to give yellow spots on pink; chloroplatinic acid with potassium iodide in acetone to give white spots on red purple; and alkaline silver nitrate. Bacillus subtilis ATCC 6633 impregnated in agar has been used to detect penicillins by observation of the zone of inhibition of the zone of ingibition after contact with the plates.

High Performance Liquid Chromatography[2] (H.P.L.C.)

HPLC method of assay reported in Indian Pharmacopeia 2007 is as following-
Buffer solution - Prepare by 0.02 M monobasic potassium phosphate solution and adjust the pH to 6.6 with 2 M sodium hydroxide.
Test solution - Weigh accurately about 55 mg of the substance under examination and dilute to 100.0 ml with the buffer solution.

Reference solution - Weigh accurately a suitable quantity of cloxacillin sodium RS, dissolve in the buffer solution and dilute to obtain a solution containing a known concentration of about 0.55 mg per ml.

Chromatographic system

A stainless steel column 25 cm x 4.6 mm, packed with octadecylsilyl silica gel 3 to 10 µm, mobile phase: a mixture of 80 volumes of the buffer solution and 20 volumes of acetonitrile, flow rate. 1 ml per minute, spectrophotometer set at 225 nm, a 20 µl loop injector. Inject the reference solution. The test is not valid unless the tailing factor is not more than 1.8 and the relative standard deviation for replicate injections is not more than 2.0 per cent. Inject alternately the test solution and the reference solution. Calculate the content of $C_{19}H_{18}ClN_3O_5S$.

Validated HPLC Method for determining cloxacillin concentration in plasma[3]

Composition of mobile phase was a mixture of 74 volumes of 100 mM potassium hydrogen phosphate solution and 26 volumes of acetonitrile. Flow rate was 1ml/minute. UV-Visible detector was set at 220 nm and a 20 µl loop injector was used. The lower limit of quantification was 0.12 µg/mL of plasma. Chromatographic system Hypersil ODS-2 column; 5 µ 250×4.6 mm.

The cloxacillin was extracted from their plasma samples by mixing the samples with precipitating agent (1% formic acid in acetonitrile) in a ratio of 1:3 v/v. The precipitated proteins were than removed by centrifugation at 3000 rpm for 10 minutes, and upper organic layer was transferred to a clean tube and dried under nitrogen flow at room temperature. The residue was reconstituted with 100 µL of mobile phase and 20 µL of aliquot was injected into chromatograph.

There are various methods reported for determining cloxacillin concentration in plasma in literature. Out of the available methods, the method described by F.W. Teare et al.[3] was found most suitable because it was practical in nature, which can be easily performed in the laboratory provided for the study.

2.1.1.4 Antimicrobial Action[4]

Cloxacillin is bactericidal with a mode of action similar to that of benzylpenicillin, but is resistant to staphylococcal penicillinase. It is active therefore against penicillinase-producing and non-penicillinase-producing staphylococci. Its activity against streptococci such as *Streptococcus pneumoniae* and *Str. pyogenes* is less than that of benzylpenicillin, but sufficient to be useful when these organisms are present with penicillin-resistant staphylococci. Cloxacillin is virtually ineffective against *Enterococcus faecalis*.

2.1.1.5 Pharmacokinetics[4]

Cloxacillin is incompletely absorbed from the gastrointestinal tract, and absorption is reduced by the presence of food in the stomach. After an oral dose of 500 mg, a peak plasma concentration of 7 to 15 micrograms/mL is attained in fasting subjects in 1 to 2 hours. Absorption is more complete when given by intramuscular injection and peak plasma concentrations of about 15 micrograms/mL have been observed 30 minutes after a dose of 500 mg. Doubling the dose can double the plasma concentration. About 94% of cloxacillin in the circulation is bound to plasma proteins. Cloxacillin has been reported to have a plasma half-life of 0.5 to 1 hour. The half-life is prolonged in neonates.

Cloxacillin crosses the placenta and is distributed into breast milk. There is little diffusion into the CSF except when the meninges are inflamed. Therapeutic concentrations can be achieved in pleural and synovial fluids and in bone.

Cloxacillin is metabolised to a limited extent, and the unchanged drug and metabolites are excreted in the urine by glomerular filtration and renal tubular secretion. About 35% of an oral dose is excreted in the urine and up to 10% in the bile. Cloxacillin is not removed by haemodialysis.

Plasma concentrations are enhanced by probenecid. Reduced concentrations in patients with cystic fibrosis have been attributed to both enhanced tubular secretion and enhanced nonrenal clearance of cloxacillin.

2.1.1.6 Uses and Administration[4]

Cloxacillin is an isoxazolyl penicillin used primarily for the treatment of infections due to staphylococci resistant to benzylpenicillin. These include bone and joint infections, endocarditis, pneumonia, skin infections (including soft-tissue infections), and toxic shock syndrome.

Cloxacillin is given by mouth as the sodium salt and doses are expressed in terms of the equivalent amount of cloxacillin. 1.09 g of cloxacillin sodium is approximately equivalent to 1 g of cloxacillin. It should be given at least 30 minutes before meals as the presence of food in the stomach reduces absorption.

Usual oral doses are 250 to 500 mg four times daily. Children may be given 50 to 100 mg/kg daily in divided doses every 6 hours.

Cloxacillin sodium has also been given by intramuscular or slow intravenous injection or infusion. Other routes of administration have included intra-articular or intrapleural injection, and inhalation.

Cloxacillin may be used with other antibacterials, including ampicillin, to produce a wider spectrum of activity. Cloxacillin benzathine is used in veterinary medicine.

2.1.2 Characterization of Cloxacillin Sodium

Cloxacillin Sodium is one of the well documented drugs; therefore, its characterization can be done with the help of experimental based on its official monograph. The procured cloxacillin sodium was characterized on the basis of pharmacopoeial monograph in I.P.

Experimental

2.1.2.1 Procurement and Identification of Cloxacillin Sodium:

Cloxacillin Sodium was obtained as gift sample from Biochem Pharmaceutical Industries ltd, Mumbai. The sample was a white crystalline powder. It was identified with the help of melting point, chemical test and its IR spectral fingerprint.

Melting Point: Melting point was determined by open capillary method in Mvtex Melting Point Apparatus. It was found 170°C with decomposition which complies with official data.

Chemical Test:

Sodium cloxacillin gave positive test for sodium salts as described in Indian Pharmacopeia. The procedure was as following-

0.1 g of the substance under examination was dissolved in 2 ml of water. 2 ml of a 15 per cent w/v solution of potassium carbonate was added and heated to boiling; no precipitate was produced. 4 ml of a freshly prepared potassium antimonate solution was added and heated to boiling. Allowed to cool in ice, a dense, white precipitate was formed.

Spectral Identification: Cloxacillin Sodium was identified by FTIR spectrophotometer. FTIR Spectrum of the Cloxacillin Sodium was recorded by FTIR spectrophotometer (Shimadzu FTIR 8400S). The recorded spectrum is shown in Figure 2.3. These spectra were matched with those shown in Figure 2.1 taken from official texts.

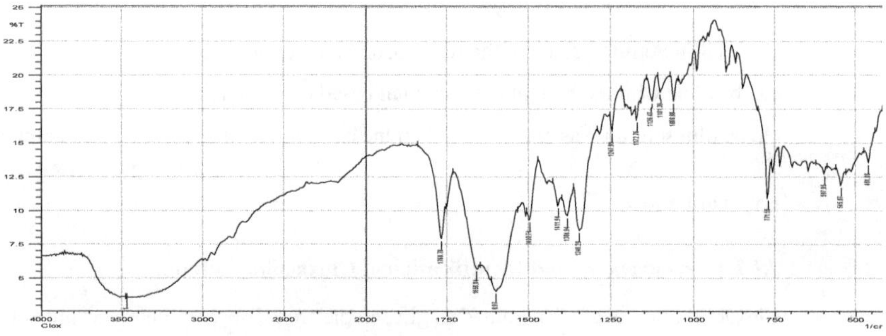

Figure 2.3: FTIR Spectrum of Cloxacillin Sodium.

2.2 CEPHALEXIN

2.2.1 Drug Profile

2.2.1.1 Description[5]

Name, Formula, Molecular Weight

Chemical Abstract designates cephalexin as 5-thia-1-azabicyclo [4, 2, 0] oct-2-ene-2-carboxylic acid, 7-(2-amino-2-phenyl-acetamido)-3-methyl-8-oxo.

Cephalexin monohydrate is also known as 5-thia-1-azabicyclo [4,2,0] oct-2-ene-2-carboxylic acid, 7-[(aminophenylacetyl) amino]-3-methyl-8-oxo, monohydrate, 7-(D-2-amino-2-phenylacetamido)-3-methyl-3-cephem-4-carboxylic acid monohydrate, and 7-(D-α-aminophenylacetamido)-3-methyl-3-cephem-4-carboxylic acid monohydrate.

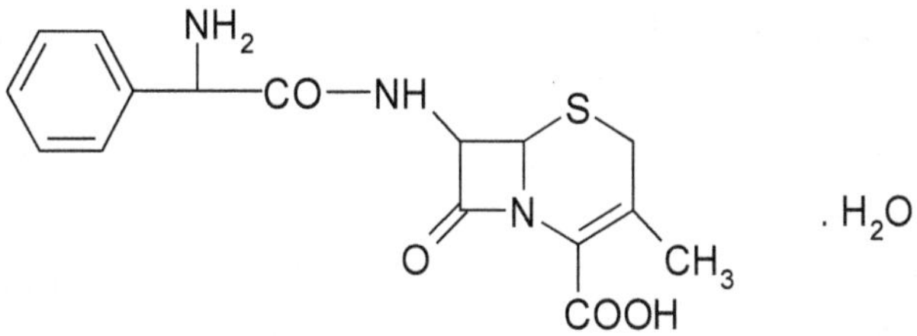

$C_{16}H_{17}N_3O_4S.H_2O$

Mol. Wt. 365.41

Isomers

The synthesis of the L epimer of cephalexin has been reported. The D-isomer exhibits considerably more biological activity than the L-isomer. Penicillins derived from D- α - amino acids also show more biological activity than their L-epimers.

Hydrates

Pfeiffer et. al. provided x-ray powder diffraction data for the monohydrate and dehydrate of cephalexin. Cephalexin was found to crystallize from aqueous solutions at room temperature as the dehydrate but converted to the mono-hydrate when the relative humidity was below 70%.

Appearance

Cephalexin is a white to cream-colored crystalline powder, having a characteristic odor.

2.2.1.2 Physical Properties[5]

Infrared Spectrum

The infrared spectrum of cephalexin monohydrate recorded as a potassium bromide disc is presented in Figure 2.4. Changes in the β-lactam carbonyl stretching region (1760 cm^{-1}) can indicate opening of the β-lactam ring. Interpretation of spectrum is as follows:

Wavelength (cm^{-1})	Assignment
3500-3000 (series of broad bands)	OH from H_2O and amide NH stretch
2600 (broad)	NH_3^+
1760	β-lactam carbonyl stretch
1690	Amide carbonyl stretch
1600 (very broad)	carboxylate stretch
820-690	Mainly skeletal vibrations including out-of-plane aromatic hydrogen bending

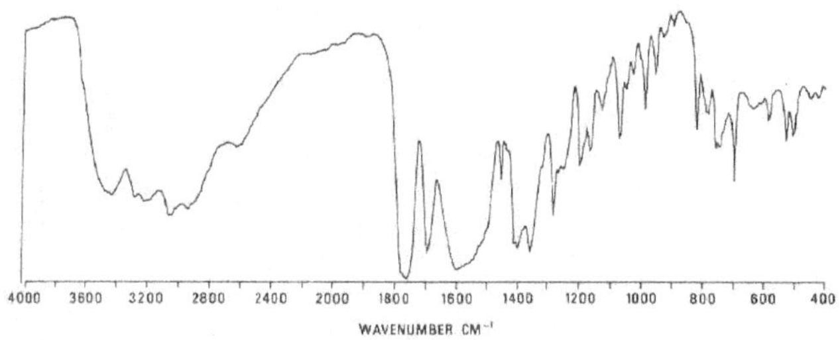

Figure 2.4 Infrared Spectrum of cephalexin monohydrate (potassium bromide disc)

Nuclear Magnetic Resonance Spectrum

Figure 2.5 shows the proton magnetic resonance spectrum of cephalexin monohydrate. The solvent used was deuterium oxide containing a small amount of trifluoroacetic acid to enhance solubility. 3-(Trimethylsilyl)-propane-sulphonic acid, sodium salt was added as the internal reference. The spectrum was recorded on a Varian T60-A instrument. The assignment of spectrum is shown as following:

Assignment	Chemical Shift, (Coupling Constant, Hz)
CH_3 (3)	2.07 s
CH_2 (2)	3.30 s
HOD (solvent)	4.85 s
H (6)	4.97 d (J=4.0)
H (benzyl)	5.34 s
H (7)	5.67 d (J=4.0)
C_6H_5	7.60 s

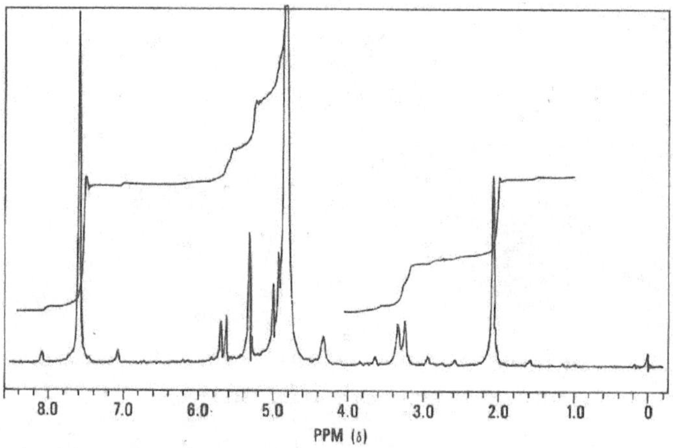

Figure 2.5 NMR spectrum of Cephalexin Monohydrate (D_2O + trifluoroacetic acid)

Crystal Properties

X-Ray Powder Diffraction

Cephalexin was found to occur in several solvated crystal forms, and often in widely varying mixtures of these forms. Some of the solvated crystals prepared were the dihydrate, monohydrate, diacetonitrilate, formamidate, methanolate, and acetonitrile hydrate.

Differential Thermal Analysis

Differential thermal analysis of cephalexin monohydrate was conducted on a DuPont Model 950 thermal analyzer in a nitrogen atmosphere. A heating rate of 20°C per minute was utilized. An endotherm was noted at 123°C indicating the loss of water, and an exotherm of 203°C indicating decomposition.

Solubility

The solubility of cephalexin monohydrate in the following solvents has been reported :

Solvent	mg. Cephalexin Monohydrate per ml. solvent, 25°C
Water	13.5
Methanol	3.4
n-Octanol	0.03
Chloroform	<0.01
Ether	<0.01

Dissociation Constant (pKa)

The following dissociation constants were reported:

	pKa	
Solvent	Carboxyl group	Amino group
66% DMF	5.2	7.3
66% DMF	5.3	7.3
H_2O	-	7.1

Optical Rotatory Dispersion

Optical rotation has been used as an auxiliary method for the quantitation of cephalexin. The specific rotation $[\alpha]_D$ reported for cephalexin, calculated on an anhydrous basis, was +153° (C= 1.0 in H_2O).

2.2.1.3 Cephalexin Stability[5]

The stability of cephalexin in solution is dependent on pH, degrading rapidly in basic media and remaining stable under mild acidic conditions. No loss in cephalexin activity occurred in 72 hours at 25° C in the pH range from 3 to 5. The rate of degradation found at pH 6 and pH 7 (25° C) was approximately 3% and 18% per day respectively. With refrigeration, no appreciable loss occured between pH 3 and pH 7 after 72 hours. In U.S.P. hydrochloric acid buffer (pH 1.2), cephalexin lost 5% activity in 24 hours at 37°C as compared to a 45% loss in phosphate buffer at pH 6.5. The antibiotic retains activity well in serum and urine as no loss in activity was noted after storage at -20° C for 14 days. Cephalexin in serum was found to lose 10%, 50% and 75% activity, respectively, after storage at 5° C, 25° C, and 37° C for 48 hours. Some organisms have been found to produce a β-lactamase (cephalosporinase) which can rapidly degrade cephalexin. Degradation of cephalexin also results from heat, strong alkali, strong acids and ultraviolet light (260 nm).

2.2.1.4 Methods of Analysis[5]

Identification Tests

Cephalexin may be identified by infrared spectroscopy. British Pharmacopoeia utilizes two characteristic color reactions for identity. Thin layer, paper, and column chromatography have been utilized for identity purposes.

Quantitative Methods:

Titration

The iodometric titration procedure has been used for the determination of cephalexin. The method is based on the fact that the intact cephalexin molecule does not consume iodine, whereas the alkali-hydrolysis product of cephalexin does. Alkaline hydrolysis of cephalexin results in cleavage of the β-lactam ring. Variations in hydrolysis time, temperature, pH of the iodine solution and concentration of cephalexin present influence the consumption of iodine by the test solution. The method compares favorably to the microbiological cylinder-plate method in accuracy, and is much more rapid. Possible intermediates used in the synthesis such as 7-ADCA will also respond to the test.

An automated iodometric assay has been used recently for the assay of cephalexin and formulations thereof. The procedure incorporates a sample hydrolysis step at 37°C for 10 minutes followed by a 5-minute iodine consumption step (pH 5.3-5.5, 37°C). Concentration of the sample is related to the decrease in iodine color measured at 350 nm. A reference standard is run concurrently through the analyzer for comparative purposes. The auto-recommended concentration range of cephalexin (0-1.5 mg. per ml. sample solution), with all standard curve plots passing through the origin. The reproducibility of the method on the same sample or standard solution on a given day is generally better than ±1% relative standard deviation (RSD). Cephalexin can be titrated with perchloric acid in a glacial acetic acid medium. Crystal violet indicator (2% in glacial acetic acid) may be used to determine the endpoint.

Moll and Doker have reported formal titration procedure for the determination of cephalexin, Ampicillin and related compounds. In this procedure 4 ml. of dilute formaldehyde solution (neutralized to the phenolphthalein end point) is added to 10 ml. of an aqueous solution containing 15.0 mg. of cephalexin. After 2 minutes the solution is titrated with 0.02N sodium hydroxide. A precision of ± 0.5% RSD would be achieved in the titration of cephalexin monohydrate raw material samples. Acidic compounds as well as amino acids must not be present as impurities in the sample. The formal titration takes advantage of the reaction between an amino acid and formaldehyde as a mean of suppressing the basicity of the amino group and thus making possible the titration of the acid.

Colorimetric Determination

Reaction with hydroxylamine has been utilized for the colorimetric determination of cephalexin. The method is based on the fact that hydroxylamine cleaves the β-lactam ring (pH 7.0) to form a hydroxamic acid which forms a colored complex with ferric ion. Degradation products or intermediates having an intact β -lactam ring react as well.

Kirschbaum has described a procedure for the colorimetric determination of the antibiotic cepharadine and related cephalosporins. An aqueous solution of the compound (1 to 30 mcg. Per ml.) is reacted with sodium hydroxide, partially neutralized, and then reacted with 5, 5'-dithiobis-(2-nitrobenzoic acid) resulting in the formation of a yellow chromophore (412 nm.). The molar absorptivity E $\times$ 10^{-4} reported for cephalexin when carried through this procedure was 1.29. The formation of the yellow chromophore was attributed to the presence of the R-$CHNH_2$-CO-cephalosporin nucleus, in which R is a mono-, di-, or tri- enyl cyclohexyl ring.

A specific colorimetric test was developed for the determination of cephalosporin derivatives having the following intact side chain in the 7-position: R- $CHNH_2$-CO-cephalosporin nucleus, R being a heterocyclic or aromatic ring. The D-phenylglycin derivatives of both 7-ADCA (cephalexin) and 7-ACA (cephaloglycin) respond well. These compounds (0.5 – 1.0 mg. per ml. in H_2O) react with acetone and sodium hydroxide at 100°C to form characteristic red chromophores (520nm). At the 1 mg. per ml. level, these tests will visually differentiate cephalexin from cephradine.

Thin Layer Chromatography

The following thin layer chromatographic systems have been reported

Adsorbent	Solvent System	R_f
Silica Gel	Acetonitrile/Water (3:1)	0.67
Silica Gel	Ethyl Acetate/Acetone/Acetic Acid/Water (5:2:2:1)	0.22
Cellulose Chromatogram Sheet	Butanol/Acetic Acid/Water (3:1:1)	-

Sheet	Ethyl Acetate/Acetic Acid/ Water (3:1:1)	-
Sheet	Acetonitrile/Ethyl Acetate/ Water (3:1:1)	-
Cellulose	Acetonitrile/Water (3:1)	0.50
Cellulose	Butanol/Acetic Acid/ Water (3:1:1)	0.70

Cellulose is the preferred sorbent since it is inert toward cephalexin. Additional thin layer chromatography systems used for cephalexin and other cephalosporins have been tabulated. Cephalexin may be detected by ultraviolet absorbance and quenching, ninhydrin, iodoplatinate, alkaline permanganate, and phosphomolybdic acid sprays.

Iodine detection and vanillin-phosphoric acid spray have also been utilized. Of the microorganisms used, Sarcina lutea is preferred over Bacillus subtilis or Staphylococcus aureus.

High Performance Liquid Chromatography[6] (H.P.L.C.)

HPLC method of assay reported in Indian Pharmacopeia 2007 is as following-

Test solution. Dissolve 50 mg of the substance under examination in water and dilute to 100.0 ml with the same solvent.

Reference solution (a). Dissolve 50 mg of cephalexin monohydrate RS in water and dilute to 100.0 ml with the same solvent.

Reference solution (b). Dissolve 10 mg of cephradine RS in 20 ml of reference solution (a) and dilute to 100 ml with water.

Chromatographic system

A stainless steel column 25 cm x 4.6 mm, packed with octadecylsilyl silica gel (5 μm), mobile phase: a mixture of 2 volumes of methanol, 5 volumes of acetonitrile, 10 volumes of a 13.6 g per liter solution of potassium dihydrogen phosphate and 83 volumes of water, flow rate. 1.5 ml per minute, spectrophotometer set at 254 nm, a 20 μl loop injector. Inject reference solution (b). In the chromatogram obtained, the resolution between the peaks due to cephalexin and cephradine is not less than 4.0. Inject alternately the test solution and reference solution (a). Calculate the content of $C_{16}H_{17}N_3O_4S$.

Validated HPLC Method for determination of cephalexin concentration in plasma[7]

Composition of mobile phase was a mixture of acetonitrile-methanol-acetate buffer of pH 4.2 (10: 10: 80 %). Flow rate was 1.4 mL/minute. UV-Visible detector was set at 254 nm and a 20 μl loop injector was used. The lower limit of quantification was 1 μg/mL of plasma. The drug was eluted from a 5 μm, C-18, reversed phase column at ambient temperature.

The cephalexin was extracted from their plasma samples by mixing the samples with precipitating agent (1% zinc sulphate solution). The precipitated proteins were than removed by centrifugation at 3000 rpm for 10 minutes, and upper organic layer was transferred to a clean tube and dried under nitrogen flow at room temperature. The residue was reconstituted with 100 μL of mobile phase and 20 μL of aliquot was injected into chromatograph.

There are various methods reported for determining cephalexin concentration in plasma in literature. Out of the available methods, the method described by N.W. Nazib et al.[7] was found most suitable because it was practical in nature, which can be easily performed in the laboratory provided for the study.

Electrophoresis

Paper electrophoresis has been utililized by the British Pharmacopoeia as a test for impurities present in cephalexin.

Microbiological Assays

Microbiological assays for cephalexin have been discussed by Marrelli, Wick, Mann, and Simmons and are listed in the Federal Register. Briefly, the two plate systems well suited for the determination of cephalexin in pharmaceutical formulations are the cylinder plate methods utilizing Staphylococcus aureus (ATCC 6535) and Bacillus subtilis (ATCC 6633). The assay range for both is approximately 2.5 to 20 mcg. of cephalexin per ml. The B. subtilis plate test has an advantage over the S. aureus plate test in that better defined zones of inhibition are obtained, thereby increasing the assay precision.

Since degradation products of cephalexin possess practically no antimicrobial activity, rapid and precise photometric microbiological assays are possible with cephalexin. The test organism for the photometric assay is Staphylococcus aureus 9144, 3 to 3.5 hours being required for incubation. If the automated AUTOTURB system used, precision in the order of 1-2% is possible. Cephalexin in biological fluids may be assayed by a Sarcina lutea plate system. The concentration range for assay is 0.2 to 3.5 mcg. /mL.

2.2.1.5 Antimicrobial Action[5]

Cefalexin is a beta-lactam antibacterial. It is bactericidal and acts similarly to benzylpenicillin by inhibiting synthesis of the bacterial cell wall. It is most active against Gram-positive cocci, and has moderate activity against some Gram-negative bacilli.

Sensitive Gram-positive cocci include both penicillinase-and non-penicillinase-producing staphylococci, although meticillin-resistant staphylococci are resistant; most streptococci are also sensitive, but not penicillin-resistant *Streptococcus pneumoniae;* enterococci are usually resistant. Some Gram-positive anaerobes are also susceptible. Cefalexin is usually inactive against *Listeria monocytogenes.*

Among Gram-negative bacteria cefalexin has activity against some Enterobacteriaceae including strains of *Escherichia coli*, *Klebsiella pneumoniae*, *Proteus mirabilis*, *Salmonella*, and *Shigella* spp., but not against *Enterobacter*, indole-positive *Proteus*, or

Serratia spp. It is also active against *Moraxella catarrhalis* (*Branhamella catarrhalis*) and *Neisseria* spp., though *Haemophilus influenzae* is moderately resistant. *Bacteroides fragilis* and *Pseudomonas aeruginosa* are not sensitive and neither are mycobacteria, mycoplasma, and fungi.

Resistance of bacteria to cefalexin may be due to several mechanisms: the drug may be prevented from reaching its site of action, for example in some Gram-negative organisms the cell wall may be a potential barrier; the target penicillin-binding proteins may be altered so that cefalexin cannot bind with these proteins; or, most importantly, the organism may produce beta-lactamases (cephalosporinases). Cefalexin is relatively resistant to hydrolysis by staphylococcal beta-lactamase, but is inactivated by a variety of beta-lactamases produced by Gram-negative organisms; resistance of Gram-negative organisms often depends on more than one factor. Resistance can be chromosomally or plasmid-mediated and may sometimes be inducible by cephalosporins.

Certain strains of bacteria may be inhibited but not killed by cephalosporins or penicillins and in such cases the minimum bactericidal concentration is much greater than the minimum inhibitory concentration; this is known as tolerance.

As well as with other cephalosporins, some cross-resistance may occur between cefalexin and the penicillinase-resistant penicillins.

Although cefalexin is generally less potent than Cefalotin. Some strains of Gram-negative bacteria may be inhibited only by the high concentrations achievable in the urinary tract. *Haemophilus influenzae* is moderately resistant to cefalexin.

2.2.1.6 Pharmacokinetics[5]

Cefalexin is almost completely absorbed from the gastrointestinal tract and produces a peak plasma concentration of about 18 micrograms/mL 1 hour after a 500-mg oral dose. If cefalexin is taken with food, absorption may be delayed, but the total amount absorbed is not appreciably altered. Up to 15% of a dose is bound to plasma proteins. The plasma half-life is about 1 hour; it increases with reduced renal function.

Cefalexin is widely distributed in the body but does not enter the CSF in significant quantities. It crosses the placenta and small quantities are found in breast milk. Cefalexin is not metabolised. About 80% or more of a dose is excreted unchanged in the urine in the first 6 hours by glomerular filtration and tubular secretion; urinary concentrations greater than 1 mg/mL have been achieved after a dose of 500 mg. Probenecid delays urinary excretion. Therapeutically effective concentrations may be found in the bile and some may be excreted by this route. Cefalexin is removed by haemodialysis and peritoneal dialysis.

2.2.1.7 Uses and Administration[8]

Cefalexin is a first-generation cephalosporin antibacterial. It is given by mouth for the treatment of susceptible infections including those of the respiratory and urinary tracts and of the skin. For severe infections, treatment with parenteral cephalosporins is to be preferred.

Cefalexin is usually given as the monohydrate although the hydrochloride is sometimes used. Doses are expressed in terms of the equivalent amount of anhydrous cefalexin. 1.05 g of cefalexin monohydrate and 1.16 g of cefalexin hydrochloride are each approximately equivalent to 1 g of anhydrous cefalexin.

The usual dose for adults is 1 to 2 g daily given in divided doses at 6-, 8-, or 12-hourly intervals; in severe or deep-seated infections the dose can be increased to up to 6 g daily but when high doses are required the use of a parenteral cephalosporin should be considered. Children may be given 25 to 100 mg/kg daily in divided doses to a maximum of 4 g daily.

For the prophylaxis of recurrent urinary-tract infection, cefalexin may be given in a dose of 125 mg at night. Cefalexin sodium or cefalexin lysine has been used parenterally.

2.2.2 Characterization of Cephalexin

Cephalexin is also a well documented drug; therefore, its characterization can be done with the help of experimental based on its official monograph. The procured cephalexin was characterized on the basis of pharmacopoeial monograph in I.P.

Experimental

Procurement and Identification of Cephalexin:

Cephalexin was purchased from Central Drug House, Delhi. The sample was a white to cream-colored crystalline powder, having a characteristic odor. It was identified with the help of melting point and its IR spectral fingerprints.

Melting Point: Melting point was determined by open capillary method in Mvtex Melting Point Apparatus. It was found 326-327°C, which complies with official data.

Spectral Identification: Cephalexin was identified by using FTIR spectrophotometer. FTIR Spectrum of the Cephalexin was recorded by FTIR spectrophotometer (Shimadzu FTIR 8400S). The recorded spectrum is shown in Figure 2.6. These spectra were matched with those shown in Figure 2.4 taken from official texts.

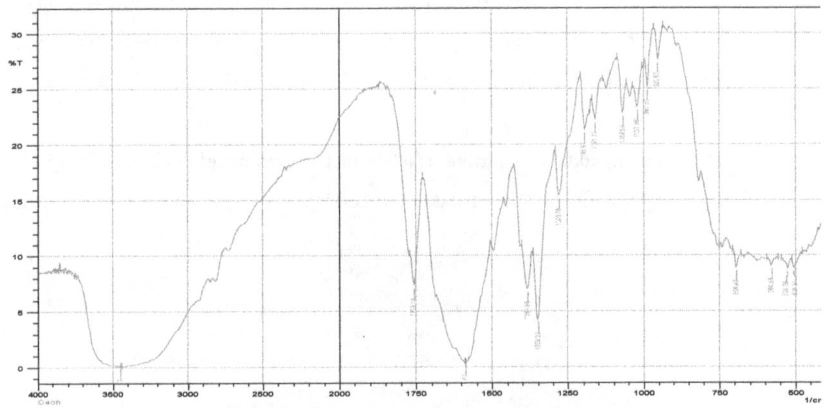

Figure 2.6: FTIR Spectrum of Cephalexin.

2.3 CIPROFLOXACIN

2.3.1 Drug Profile

2.3.1.1 Description[9]

Name, Formula, Molecular Weight

1-Cyclopropyl-6-fluoro-1, 4-dihydro-4-oxo-7-(1-piperazinyl)-3-quinolinecarboxylic acid.

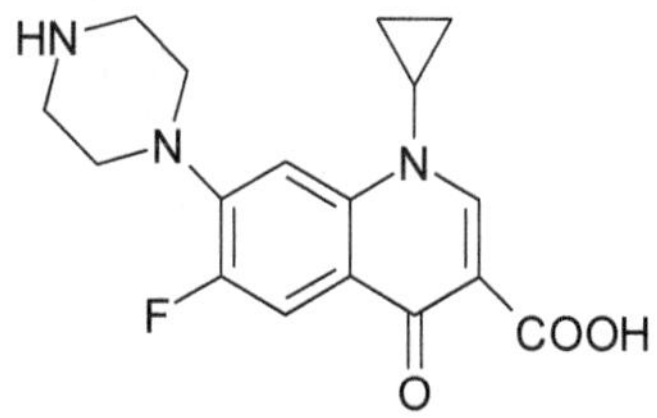

$C_{17}H_{18}FN_3O_3$ Mol. Wt. = 331.35

Appearance

Ciprofloxacin is obtained as a light yellow crystalline powder.

2.3.1.2 Physical Properties[9]

Infrared spectrum

The infrared absorption spectrum of ciprofloxacin was obtained in a KBr pellet using Perkin Elmer infrared spectrophotometer. The infrared spectrum is shown in Figure 2.7 and the assignments for the major infrared absorption bands are as following:

Frequency (cm-1)	Assignment
3490	O-H stretch
3320	N-H stretch of piperazinyl moiety
2930	Aliphatic C-H stretch
1696	C=O stretch of carboxyl group
1605	C=O stretch of quinoline carboxyl

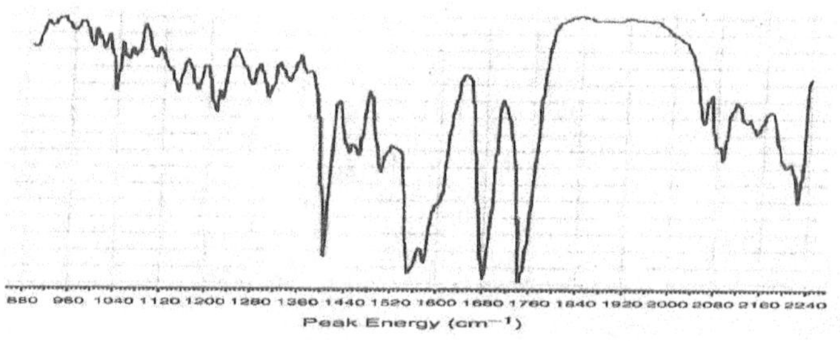

Figure 2.7 Infrared spectrum of ciprofloxacin

Nuclear Magnetic Resonance spectrum

The proton NMR spectrum of ciprofloxacin was obtained using a Bruker Advance system, operating at 300, 400 and 500 MHz. The sample was dissolved in D_2O and tetramethylsilane (TMS) was used as the internal standard. The proton NMR spectrum is shown in Fig. 2.8 and assignments for the proton NMR bands of ciprofloxacin are found as follow:

Assignment	Chemical Shift, (Coupling Constant, Hz)
H-2	8.63 s
H-5	7.46 d
H-8	7.52 d
H-2', 6' or 3', 5'	3.66 d
H-1a	1.22 s
H-1b, 1c	1.47 d

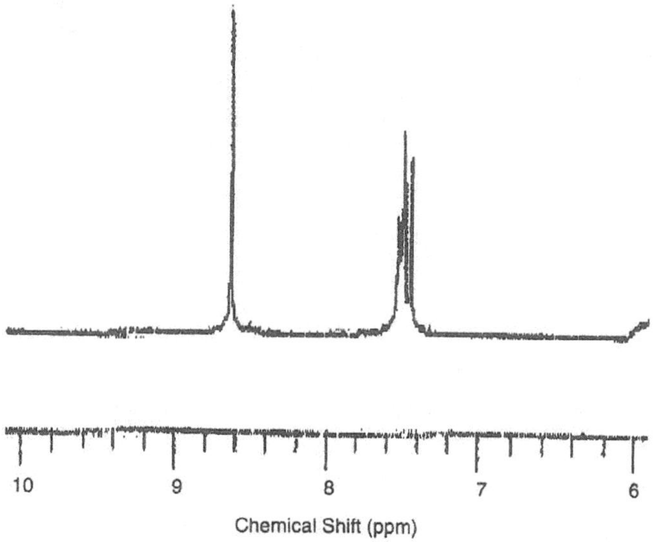

Figure 2.8 H[1]-NMR spectrum of ciprofloxacin in D_2O

Solubility characteristics

Ciprofloxacin is practically insoluble in water, very slightly soluble in dehydrated alcohol & dichloromethane, and soluble in dilute acetic acid.

Optical activity

Since ciprofloxacin has no centers of dissymmetry, it does not exhibit optical activity.

2.3.1.3 Stability and storage[9]

Solutions of ciprofloxacin are light sensitive and should be protected from light and freezing. When the concentrate formulated for intravenous injection, or the 1.2 g pharmacy bulk package, is diluted with 5% dextrose injection or 0.9% sodium chloride injection to a final concentration of 0.5-2 mg/ml, the resultant solution is stable for upto 14 days when stored at room temperature or when refrigerated at 2-8° C.

The commercially available injection for intravenous infusion that contains 2 mg/mL in 5% dextrose is provided in a plastic container fabricated from a specially formulated polyvinyl chloride (PVC). Tammilehto et al. used thin-layer chromatography to study the degradation of ciprofloxacin hydrochloride solutions after these were irradiated by a high pressure mercury lamp.

2.3.1.4 Reported Methods of Analysis[9]

Identification

The European Pharmacopoeia recommends the use of infrared absorption spectrophotometry for the identification of the pure drug substance. The procedure entails an examination by infrared absorption spectrophotometry, and a comparison with the spectrum obtained with the ciprofloxacin reference standard.

Quantitative Methods

Titration Method

Four DNA topoisomerase inhibitors, including ciprofloxacin (alone or in mixture with other drugs), were determined by a titration method. Tablets containing ciprofloxacin were extracted three times with 30 mL of methanol. A portion of the resulting solution was mixed with 2 mL water, and that solution was titrated with aqueous 5mM NaOH,

5mM tetrabutyl-ammonium hydroxide, or 5 mM $AgNO_3$ by adding 0.1 mL increments at 2 min intervals. The end-point was detected using the solution conductance.

Spectrophotometric method

Rizk et al[9]. developed a sensitive and selective derivative UV-spectrophotometric method for the determination of three fluoroquinolone compounds, including ciprofloxacin, in formulations and spiked biological fluids. The method depends on the complexation of Cu (II) with the studied compounds in an aqueous medium. A linear correlation was established between the amplitude of the peak and the drug concentration over the range of 35-120 ng/mL. The detection limit was reported as 1.3 ng/mL. The method was used for the determination of the ciprofloxacin bulk drug substance and its tablet formulation, with an overall percentage recovery of 99.22±0.55 to 100.33±1.60.

Chemiluminescence method

Aly et al[9]. reported a rapid and sensitive chemiluminescence (CL) method for the determination of three fluoroquinolone derivatives, including ciprofloxacin, in both pharmaceutical dosage forms and in biological fluids. The method is based on the CL reaction of the drugs with tris (2,2'-bipyridyl)ruthenium(II) and cerium(IV) in sulfuric acid medium. The CL intensity was proportional to the concentration of ciprofloxacin in solution over the range 0.05-6 μg/mL, and the limit of detection was reported to be 26 nM.

Electrochemical methods

The voltammetric behavior of the Ni (II) complexes of three 4-quinolone antibacterial compounds in tablets, including ciprofloxacin, was studied using direct current (Dct), differential pulse (DPP) and alternating current polarography (Act). A well defined, cathodic wave was detected at pH 5.5 for ciprofloxacin. The current-concentration relationship was found to be linear over the range $2 - 6.4 \times 10^{-5}$ M and $0.8 - 5.6 \times 10^{-5}$ M for ciprofloxacin using DCt and DPP modes, respectively. Limits of detection (S/N=2) for these species were found to be about 2×10^{-7}M. The average percent recovery for ciprofloxacin was 99.58±0.72 to 100.50±0.79, and 99.50±0.71 to 100.17±0.29, when using DCt and DPP, respectively.

Thin layer chromatography

Mixtures of antibacterial agents (including ciprofloxacin hydrochloride) together with p-aminophenol (internal standard) in 0.1 M HCl were analyzed by thin layer chromatography (TLC). The system used a silica gel GF254 plate and a mobile phase consisting of chloroform/methanol/concentrated ammonium hydroxide (15:10:3). The chromatogram was examined under a UV lamp at 254 nm, and it was found that all spots were cleanly separated.

High Performance liquid chromatographic method[10]

HPLC method of assay reported in Indian Pharmacopeia (2007) is as following-

Test solution. Weigh accurately about 25 mg, add 0.2 ml of a solution containing 7 per cent v/v of phosphoric acid and add sufficient of the mobile phase to produce 50.0 ml.
Reference solution (a).Prepare in the same manner as the test solution using an accurately weighed quantity of ciprofloxacin RS in place of the substance under examination.
Reference solution (b). A 0.05 per cent w/v solution of ciprofloxacin ethylenediamine analog RS in reference solution (a).
Chromatographic system
a stainless steel column 25 cm × 4 mm, packed with octadecylsilyl silica gel (5 µm), mobile phase: a mixture of 87 volumes of 0.025 M phosphoric acid, previously adjusted with triethylamine to a pH of 3.0 ± 0.1, and 13 volumes of acetonitrile, flow rate. 1.5 ml per minute, column temperaure. 30° ± 1°, spectrophotometer set at 278 nm, a 10 µl loop injector.

Inject reference solution (b) and record the chromatogram adjusting the sensitivity and flow rate suitably so that the retention time for ciprofloxacin is between 6.4 and 10.8 minutes, the relative retention times are about 0.7 for ciprofloxacin ethylenediamine analog and 1.0 for ciprofloxacin and the resolution between ciprofloxacin ethylenediamine analog peak and ciprofloxacin peak is not less than 6. The column efficiency, determined from ciprofloxacin peak, is not less than 2500 theoretical plates, the tailing factor for the ciprofloxacin peak is not more than 4.0 and the relative standard deviation for replicate injections is not more than 1.5 per cent. Inject alternately the test solution and reference solution (a). Calculate the content of $C_{17}H_{18}FN_3O_3$.

Validated HPLC Method for determining ciprofloxacin concentration in plasma[11]

Composition of mobile phase was a mixture of 0.01 M phosphate buffer (pH = 2.6, adjusted with concentrated orthophosphoric acid) and methanol in a ratio of 82 and 18 v/v respectively. Flow rate was 1.5 mL/minute. UV-Visible detector was set at 277 nm and a 20 µl loop injector was used. The lower limit of quantification was 20 ng/mL of plasma. Separation was carried on a Novapak C 18 column.

The ciprofloxacin was extracted from their plasma samples by mixing the samples with precipitating agent (1% formic acid in acetonitrile) in a ratio of 1:3 v/v. The precipitated proteins were than removed by centrifugation at 3000 rpm for 10 minutes, and upper organic layer was transferred to a clean tube and dried under nitrogen flow at room temperature. The residue was reconstituted with 100 µL of mobile phase and 20 µL of aliquot was injected into chromatograph.

There are various methods reported for determining ciprofloxacin concentration in plasma in literature, out of the available methods, the method described by M. Amini et al.[11] was found most suitable because it was practical in nature, which can be easily performed in the laboratory provided for the study.

Gas chromatography

Gas chromatography was used to analyze the residual piperazine of ciprofloxacin and norfloxacin in pharmaceutical preparations. The analyte was dissolved in water, and the solution analyzed by GC on a fused silica column (30 m × 0.3 mm i.d.) coated with 5% cross linked ph-Me silicone (3 μm). The temperature Programme consisted of an increase to 50° C, holding for 5 min, ramping to 180° C (ramp = 15°C/min), and finally holding for 10 min at 180°C (5°C /min). Nitrogen was used as the carrier gas (flow rate of 1ml/min), detection was effected using flame ionization. Piperazine was determined in the two mixtures by mixing for 10 min with cyclohexane, filtering, partitioning the filtrate with water, heating the aqueous phase at 45° C for 10 min, and then analyzing as above. The calibration graph was linear for 0.4-10 ppm piperazine, with a RSD (n =10) of 2.1% for 2μg piperazine. The recovery from ciprofloxacin was 98.1-98.4%.

2.3.1.5 Antimicrobial Action[9]

Ciprofloxacin is bactericidal and acts by inhibiting the A subunit of DNA gyrase (topoisomerase) which is essential in the reproduction of bacterial DNA. It has a broader spectrum of activity and is more potent *in vitro* than the non-fluorinated quinolone nalidixic acid. Activity may be reduced in acid media.

Spectrum of activity. Among Gram-negative aerobic bacteria, ciprofloxacin is active *in vitro* against Enterobacteriaceae, including *Escherichia coli* and *Citrobacter*, *Enterobacter*, *Klebsiella*, *Proteus*, *Providencia*, *Salmonella*, *Serratia*, *Shigella*, and *Yersinia* spp. It is also active against *Pseudomonas aeruginosa*, but less so against other *Pseudomonas* spp. *Haemophilus ducreyi*, *H. influenzae*, *Moraxella catarrhalis* (*Branhamella catarrhalis*), and *Neisseria gonorrhoeae* are all very sensitive, including beta-lactamase-producing strains; *N. meningitidis* is also susceptible. Other Gram-negative aerobic bacteria reported to be sensitive to ciprofloxacin have included *Acinetobacter* spp., *Campylobacter* spp., *Gardnerella vaginalis*, *Helicobacter pylori*,

Legionella spp., *Pasteurella multocida*, and *Vibrio* spp. Variable activity has been reported against *Brucella melitensis*.

Among Gram-positive aerobic bacteria, ciprofloxacin is active against staphylococci, including penicillinase-producing and penicillinase-nonproducing strains, and against some meticillin-resistant strains. Streptococci, in particular *Streptococcus pneumoniae* and enterococci, are less susceptible. Other Gram-positive bacteria sensitive to ciprofloxacin *in vitro* are *Bacillus anthracis* and *Corynebacterium* spp.

Most anaerobic bacteria, including *Bacteroides fragilis* and *Clostridium difficile*, are resistant to ciprofloxacin, although some other *Clostridium* spp. may be susceptible.

Ciprofloxacin has some activity against mycobacteria, mycoplasmas, rickettsias, and the protozoan *Plasmodium falciparum*. *Chlamydia trachomatis* is moderately susceptible, and *Nocardia asteroides* and *Ureaplasma urealyticum* are usually considered to be resistant. The spirochaete *Treponema pallidum* and fungi are also resistant.

Activity with other antimicrobials. There have been some reports of enhanced activity *in vitro* when ciprofloxacin has been used with other antimicrobials, such as aminoglycosides or azlocillin against *Staphylococcus aureus* and *Pseudomonas aeruginosa*, imipenem against *Ps. aeruginosa*, and cefotaxime or clindamycin against anaerobic bacteria.

Acquired resistance. Resistant strains, particularly of *Staph. aureus* (including meticillin-resistant strains) and *Ps. aeruginosa* have emerged during treatment with ciprofloxacin. There is complete cross-resistance between ciprofloxacin and the other fluoroquinolones, but not between ciprofloxacin and nalidixic acid. Like nalidixic acid, resistance to ciprofloxacin appears, so far, to be chromosomally rather than plasmid-mediated.

2.3.1.6 Pharmacokinetics[9]

Ciprofloxacin is rapidly and well absorbed from the gastrointestinal tract. Oral bioavailability is approximately 70% and a peak plasma concentration of about 2.5 micrograms/mL is achieved 1 to 2 hours after a dose of 500 mg by mouth. Absorption may be delayed by the presence of food, but is not substantially affected overall. The plasma half-life is about 3.5 to 4.5 hours and there is evidence of modest accumulation. Half-life may be prolonged in renal impairment—a value of 8 hours has been reported in end-stage renal disease—and to some extent in the elderly. There is limited information on the effect of hepatic impairment; the half-life of ciprofloxacin has been reported to be slightly prolonged in patients with severe cirrhosis of the liver. With one or two exceptions, most studies have shown the pharmacokinetics of ciprofloxacin to be not markedly affected by cystic fibrosis.

Plasma protein binding ranges from 20 to 40%. Ciprofloxacin is widely distributed in the body and tissue penetration is generally good. It appears in the CSF, but concentrations are only about 10% of those in plasma when the meninges are not inflamed. Ciprofloxacin crosses the placenta and is also distributed into breast milk. High concentrations are achieved in bile.

Ciprofloxacin is eliminated principally by urinary excretion, but non-renal clearance may account for about a third of elimination and includes hepatic metabolism, biliary excretion, and possibly transluminal secretion across the intestinal mucosa. At least 4 active metabolites have been identified. Oxociprofloxacin appears to be the major urinary metabolite and sulfociprofloxacin the primary faecal metabolite. Urinary excretion is by active tubular secretion as well as glomerular filtration and is reduced by probenecid; it is virtually complete within 24 hours. About 40 to 50% of an oral dose is excreted unchanged in the urine and about 15% as metabolites. Up to 70% of a parenteral dose may be excreted unchanged within 24 hours and 10% as metabolites. Faecal excretion over 5 days has accounted for 20 to 35% of an oral dose and 15% of an intravenous dose. Only small amounts of ciprofloxacin are removed by haemodialysis or peritoneal dialysis.

2.3.1.7 Uses and Administration[12]

Ciprofloxacin is a fluorinated 4-quinolone or fluoroquinolone antibacterial with a wider spectrum of activity than nalidixic acid and more favourable pharmacokinetics allowing its use in systemic infections. It has been used in the treatment of a wide range of infections including anthrax, biliary-tract infections, infected bites and stings, bone and joint infections, cat scratch disease, chancroid, exacerbations of cystic fibrosis, gastro-enteritis (including travellers' diarrhoea and campylobacter enteritis, cholera, salmonella enteritis, and shigellosis), gonorrhoea, infections in immunocompromised patients (neutropenia), legionnaires' disease, otitis externa, otitis media, peritonitis, Q fever, lower respiratory-tract infections (including pseudomonal infections in cystic fibrosis, but excluding infections due to *Streptococcus pneumoniae* such as pneumococcal pneumonia), septicaemia, skin infections (including soft-tissue infections), spotted fevers, typhoid and paratyphoid fever, typhus, and urinary-tract infections. Ciprofloxacin is used for meningococcal meningitis prophylaxis. It is also used for surgical infection prophylaxis. Fluoroquinolones such as ciprofloxacin and ofloxacin have been tried in the treatment of opportunistic mycobacterial infections and tuberculosis; ofloxacin may be used in the treatment of leprosy. Fluoroquinolones such as ciprofloxacin and ofloxacin are used topically in the treatment of eye infections.

2.3.1.8 Administration and dosage[12]

Ciprofloxacin is given by mouth as the hydrochloride or base, by intravenous infusion as the lactate, and in eye drops or eye ointment as the hydrochloride. Doses and strengths are expressed in terms of the equivalent amount of ciprofloxacin base. 291.1 mg of ciprofloxacin hydrochloride is approximately equivalent to 250 mg of ciprofloxacin. 127 mg of ciprofloxacin lactate is approximately equivalent to 100 mg of ciprofloxacin.

The usual adult oral dose of ciprofloxacin ranges from 250 to 750 mg twice daily depending on the severity and nature of the infection. The usual adult intravenous dose is 100 to 400 mg twice daily, given over 30 to 60 minutes as a solution containing the equivalent of 1 to 2 mg/mL. A dose of 100 mg twice daily by mouth is suitable in women with acute uncomplicated cystitis.

For acute exacerbations of cystic fibrosis associated with *Pseudomonas aeruginosa* infection, ciprofloxacin may be given to adolescents and children aged 5 years or more in a dose of 20 mg/kg by mouth twice daily, up to a maximum of 750 mg twice daily. Alternatively, a dose of 10 mg/kg may be given by intravenous infusion over 60 minutes three times daily, to a maximum of 400 mg three times daily.

For inhalation anthrax, ciprofloxacin may be given to children and adolescents for 60 days in a dose of 15 mg/kg twice daily by mouth, up to a maximum of 500 mg twice daily. Alternatively, a dose of 10 mg/kg twice daily may be given by intravenous infusion, up to a maximum of 400 mg twice daily.

Ciprofloxacin is not generally recommended for other uses in children and adolescents but, if considered essential, doses of 5 to 15 mg/kg twice daily by mouth or 4 to 8 mg/kg twice daily intravenously have been suggested.

Doses should be reduced in patients with severe renal impairment.

Single oral doses of 250 or 500 mg are used for the treatment of gonorrhoea, depending upon patterns of resistance. A single oral dose of 500 mg is suggested for meningococcal meningitis prophylaxis. A single oral dose of 750 mg is suggested for surgical infection prophylaxis, given 60 to 90 minutes before the procedure.

For corneal ulcers and superficial ocular infections caused by susceptible strains of bacteria ciprofloxacin is given as the hydrochloride in eye drops and eye ointment containing the equivalent of 0.3% of ciprofloxacin base.

2.3.2 Characterization of Ciprofloxacin

Ciprofloxacin is one of the best documented drugs; therefore, its characterization can be done with the help of experimental based on its official monograph. The procured ciprofloxacin was characterized on the basis of pharmacopeial monograph in I.P.

Experimental

Procurement and Identification of Ciprofloxacin:

Ciprofloxacin was purchased from Central Drug House, Delhi. The sample was a light yellow crystalline powder. It was identified with the help of melting point and its IR spectral fingerprints.

Melting Point: Melting point was determined by open capillary method in Mvtex Melting Point Apparatus. It was found 318-320°C, which complies with official data.

Spectral Identification: Ciprofloxacin was identified by using FTIR spectrophotometer. FTIR Spectrum of the Ciprofloxacin was recorded by FTIR spectrophotometer (Shimadzu FTIR 8400S). The recorded spectrum is shown in Figure 2.9. These spectra were matched with those shown in Figure 2.7 taken from official texts.

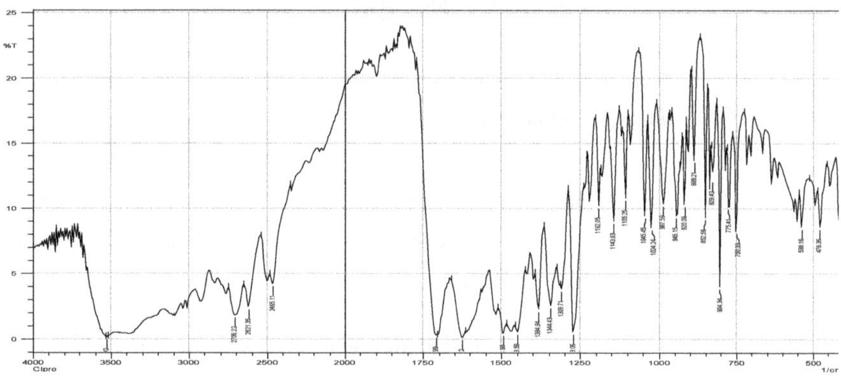

Figure 2.9: FTIR Spectrum of Ciprofloxacin.

REFERENCES

1. L.M. David, Cloxacillin Sodium, Analytical Profiles of Drug Substances, vol. 4, Florey, Academic Press, An imprint of Elsevier, 1975, 113-136.

2. Cloxacillin, Indian Pharmacopoeia 2007, vol. 2, Government of India, Ministry of Health & Family Welfare, Published by the Indian Pharmacopoeia Commission, Ghaziabad, 2007, 960.

3. Teare FW, Kwan RH, Spino M, Macleod SM. High-pressure liquid chromatographic assay of cloxacillin in serum and urine. J Pharm Sci. 71, 938-941 (1982).

4. Cloxacillin, Martindale, The Complete drug Reference, 36th Edition, Sweetman, Published by Pharmaceutical Press, 2009, vol. 1, 256.

5. P.M. Louis, Cephalexin, Analytical Profiles of Drug Substances, vol. 4, Florey, Academic Press, An imprint of Elsevier, 1975, 21-46.

6. Cephalexin, Indian Pharmacopoeia 2007, vol. 2, Government of India, Ministry of Health & Family Welfare, Published by the Indian Pharmacopoeia Commission, Ghaziabad, 2007, 886.

7. Najib NW et al. High Performance liquid chromatographic analysis of cephalexin in serum and urine. Journal of Clinical Pharmacy and Therapeutics; 12, 419-426 (1987).

8. Cephalexin, Martindale, The Complete drug Reference, 36th Edition, Sweetman, Published by Pharmaceutical Press, 2009, vol. 1, 218-19.

9. Al-omar M.A., Ciprofloxacin, Profiles of Drug Substances, Excipients, and Related Methodology, vol. 31, Brittain, Academic Press, An imprint of Elsevier, 2004, 163-214.

10. Ciprofloxacin, Indian Pharmacopoeia 2007, vol. 2, Government of India, Ministry of Health & Family Welfare, Published by the Indian Pharmacopoeia Commission, Ghaziabad, 2007, 936.

11. Amini M.; Khanavi M; Shafiee A; Simple High Performance Liquid Chromatographic Method for Determination of Ciprofloxacin in Human Plasma. Iranian Journal of Pharmaceutical Research 2, 99-101 (2004).

12. Ciprofloxacin, Martindale, The Complete drug Reference, 36th Edition, Sweetman, Published by Pharmaceutical Press 2009, vol.1, 246-47.

SYNTHESES (DRUG DERIVATIZATION)

General Methods of Dendrimer Synthesis

Dendrimers can be considered to have three major portions: a core, an inner shell, and an outer shell. Ideally a dendrimer can be synthesized to have different functionality in each of these portions to control properties such as solubility, thermal stability, and attachment of compounds for particular application. Synthetic processes can also precisely control the size and number of branches on the dendrimer. There are two defined methods of dendrimer synthesis, divergent synthesis and convergent synthesis. The first dendrimers were made by divergent synthesis approaches by Fritz Vögtle in 1978,[1] R.G. Denkewalter at Allied Corporation in 1981,[2,3] Donald Tomalia at Dow Chemical in 1983[4] and in 1985,[5,6] and by George Newkome in 1985.[7] In 1990 a convergent synthetic approach was introduced by Jean Fréchet.[8]

Divergent Methods

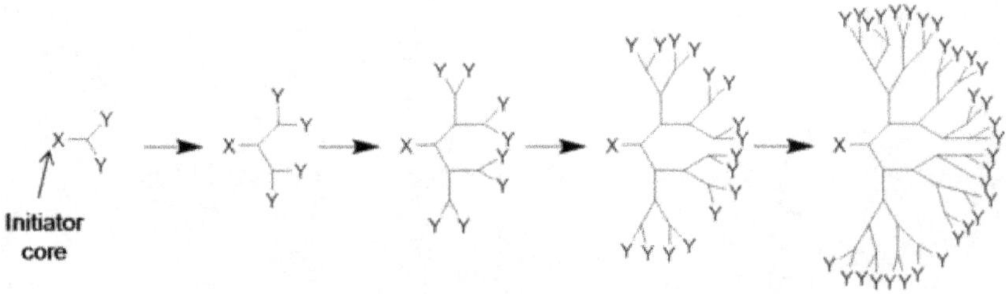

Figure 3.1: Schematic of divergent synthesis of dendrimers

The dendrimer is assembled from a multifunctional core, which is extended outward by a series of reactions, commonly a Michael reaction. Each step of the reaction must be driven to full completion to prevent mistakes in the dendrimer, which can cause trailing generations (some branches are shorter than the others). Such impurities can impact the functionality and symmetry of the dendrimer, but are extremely difficult to purify out because the relative size difference between perfect and imperfect dendrimers is very small.

Convergent Methods

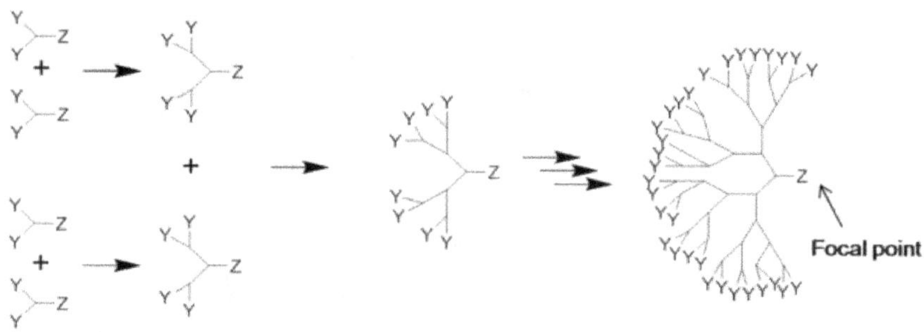

Figure 3.2: Schematic of convergent synthesis of dendrimers

Dendrimers are built from small molecules that end up at the surface of the sphere, and reactions proceed inward building inward and are eventually attached to a core. This method makes it much easier to remove impurities and shorter branches along the way, so that the final dendrimer is more monodisperse. However dendrimers made this way are not as large as those made by divergent methods because crowding due to steric effects along the core is limiting.

Selection of Method for Dendrimer Synthesis

There are mainly two methods divergent and convergent for dendrimer synthesis. Main disadvantage of convergent method is that we cannot synthesize a large molecule for drug loading due to crowding and steric effect as shown in fig. 3.2. Hence divergent method of dendrimer synthesis was selected.

3.1 Scheme of Synthesis

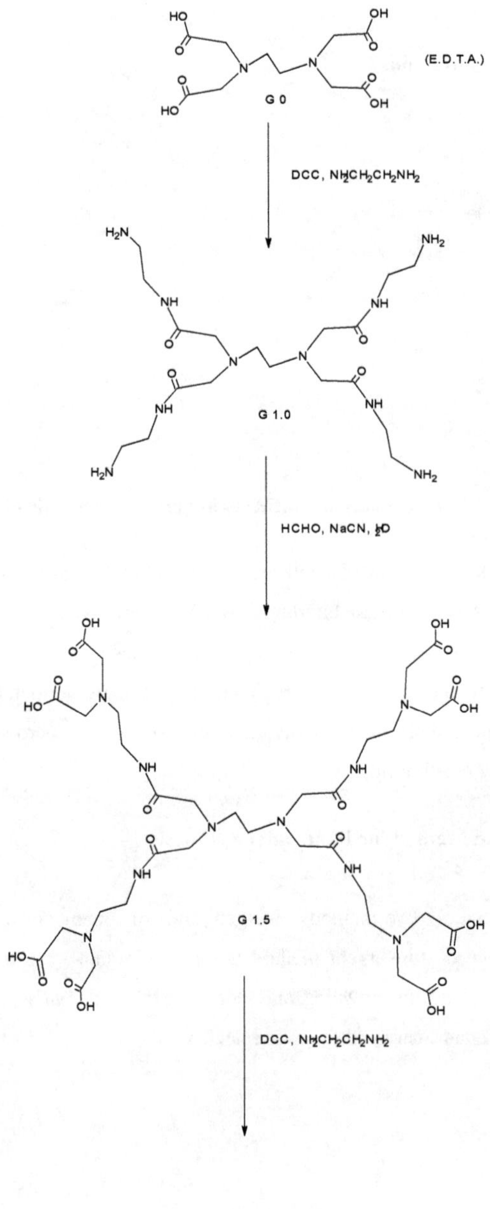

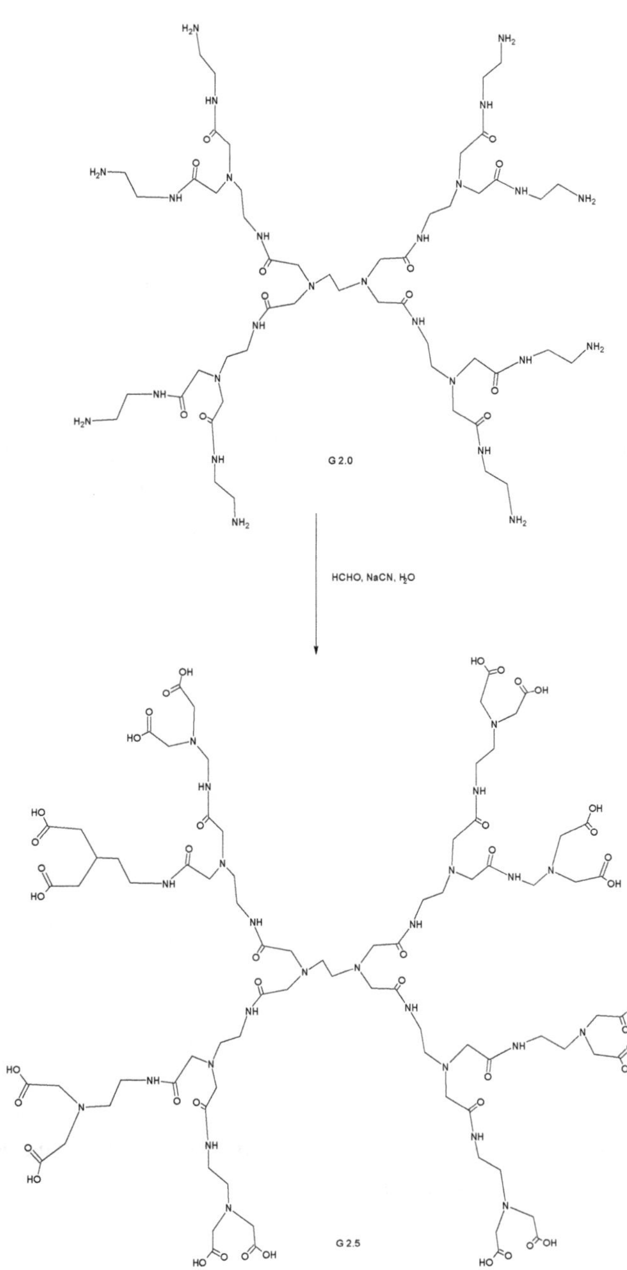
G 2.0
HCHO, NaCN, H_2O
G 2.5

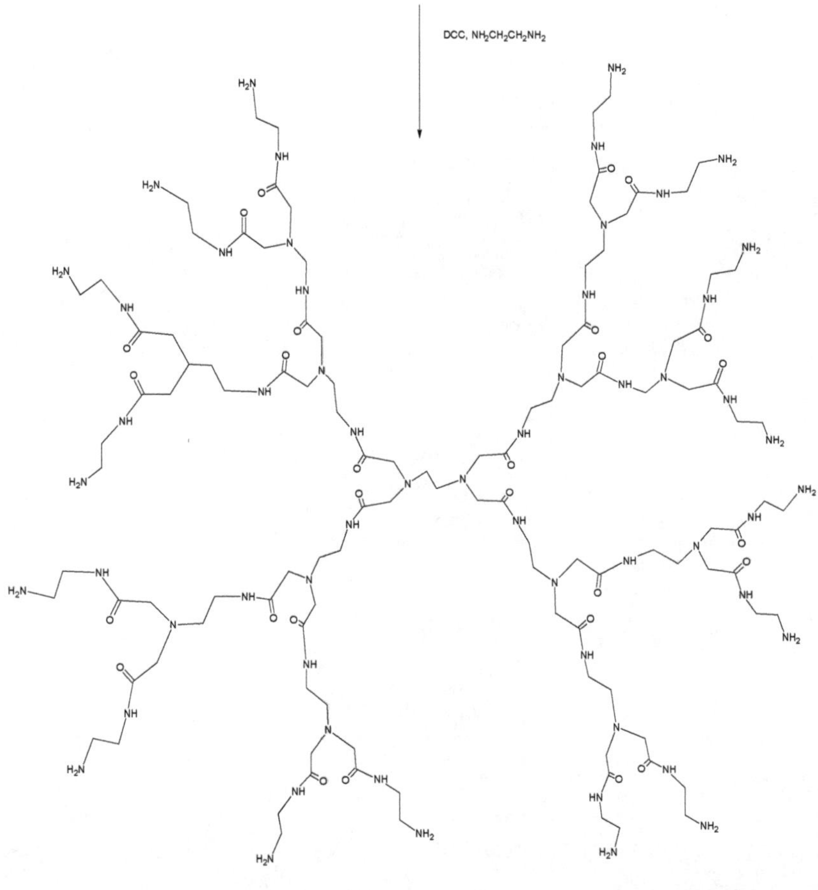

Scheme 1. Synthesis of EDTA core PAMAM dendrimer (G 3.0) having 16 free primary amine groups

Chemical Loading of Drugs on PEG 4000

After synthesis of dendrimer, PEGylated drug molecules were synthesized following general procedure given by Zilipsky et. al.[9] and is described in scheme 2.

PEGylated Drug Molecules Loading on Dendrimer

After synthesis of PEGylated drug molecules, they are conjugated with terminal NH_2 groups of PAMAM dendrimer, so that final drug-conjugated PEG-PAMAM star polymers could be synthesized (Figure 3.3, 3.4 and 3.5). The synthetic scheme for the same is described in scheme 2.

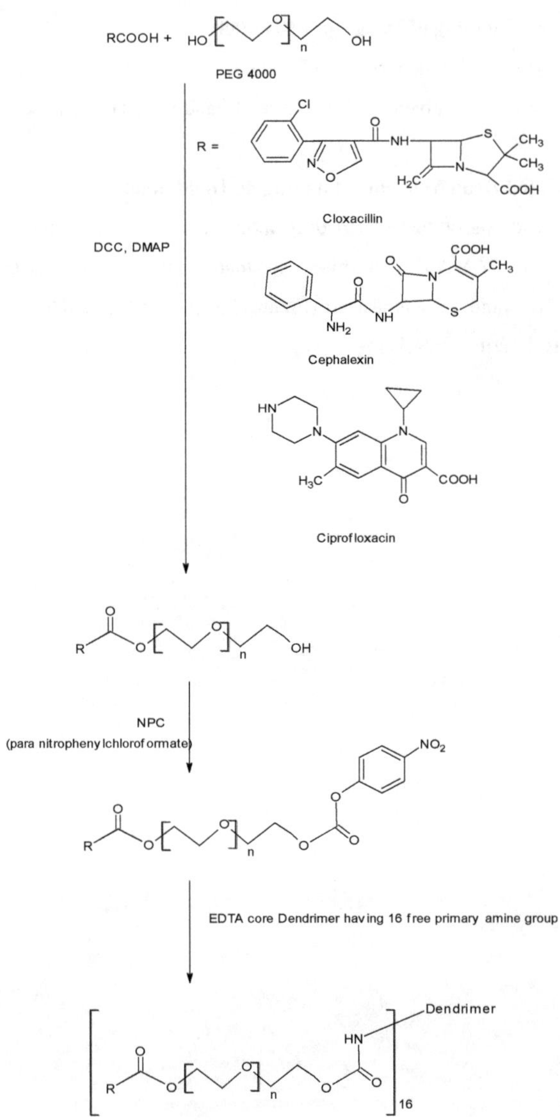

Scheme 2. Synthesis of drug-PEG 4000-dendrimer complex

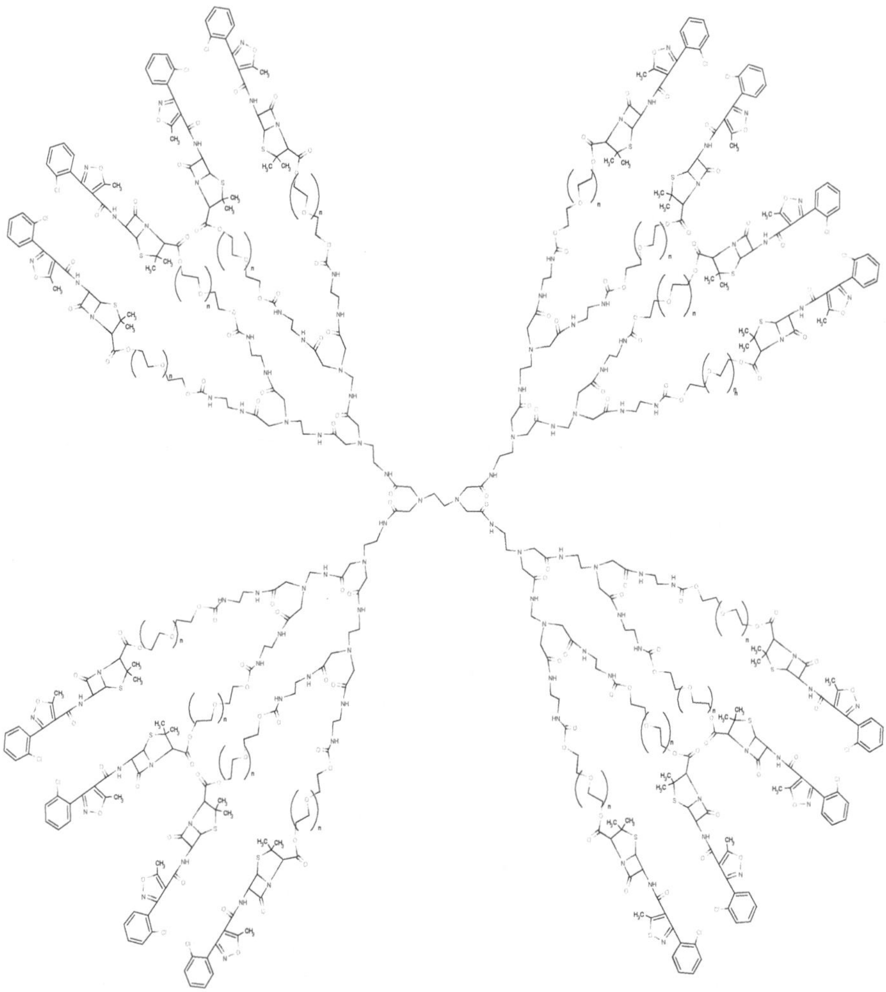

Figure 3.3. Idealized schematic view of drug contained poly ethylene glycol star polymer. PAMAM dendrimer with EDTA core contains 16 primary amino groups which connect MW 4000 poly ethylene glycol; Cloxacillin is attached to the end of PEG (Structure of final derivatized cloxacillin)

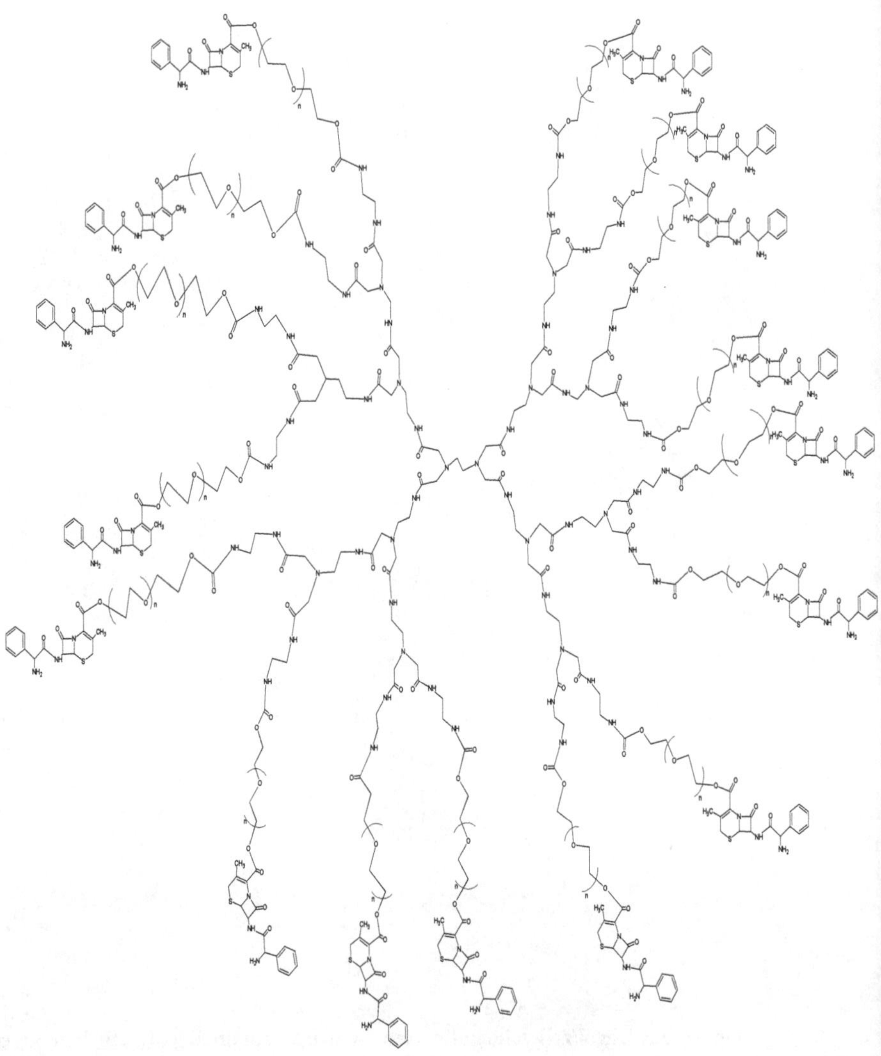

Figure 3.4 Structure of final derivatized cephalexin

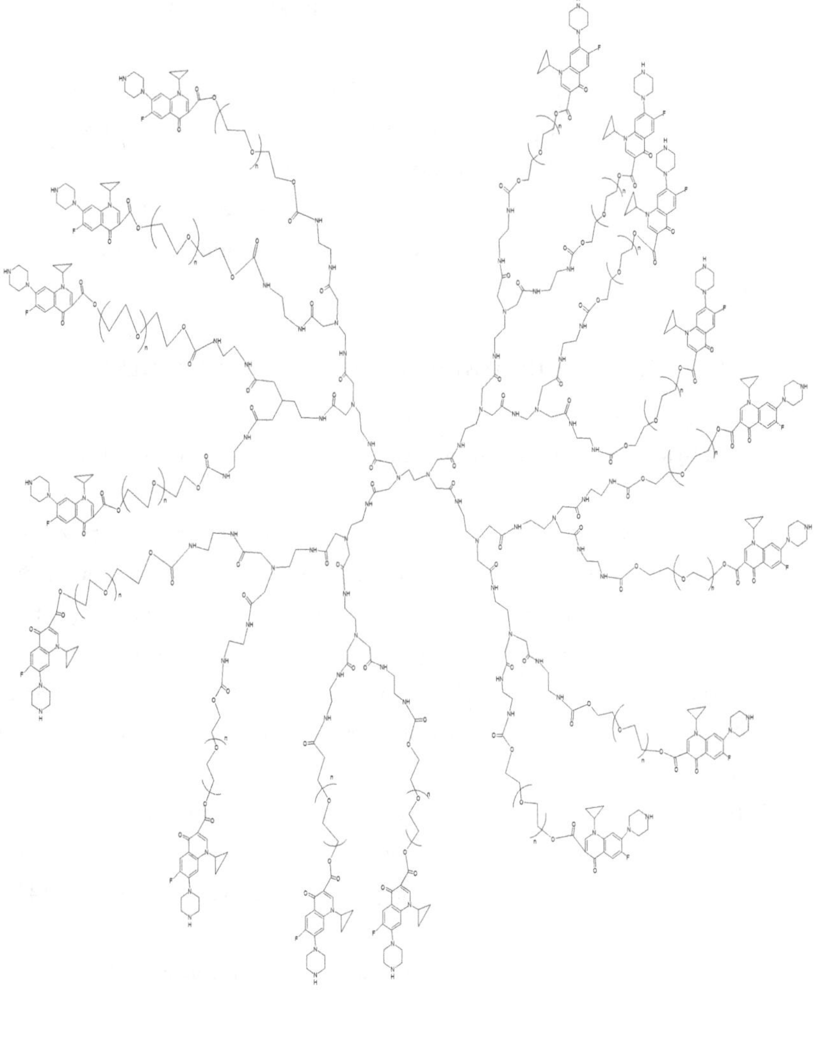

Figure 3.5 Structure of final derivatized ciprofloxacin

3.2 SYNTHESIS OF NOVEL EDTA CORE BASED DENDRIMER

Present dendrimer was synthesized using EDTA as a core or starting material having four carboxylic groups for growth. EDTA was reacted with ethylenediamine in presence of DCC in first step. Then the product of first step was reacted with sodium cyanide & formaldehyde in second step. Then these two steps were repeated to form dendrimer having 16 free $-NH_2$ groups on surface (Scheme 1). Dendrimer and its intermediates were characterized by FTIR & H^1-NMR analysis.

3.3 SYNTHESIS OF CLOXACILLIN-CONJUGATED PEG-DENDRIMER (C-3)

3.3.1 Synthesis of Cloxacillin conjugated PEG 4000 (C-1) via ester bond:

The synthesis was carried out following the general procedure given by Zalipsky et al[9] (Scheme 2). 1.2 mmole (523 mg) of cloxacillin was dissolved in 50 ml of dichloromethane and cooled in ice bath (0°C). Then 1.3 mmole (268.2g) of DCC was added to solution with stirring. Then 1.2 mmole (146.6g) of DMAP (4-dimethylaminopyridine) was added to the reaction mixture. After this addition 2 mmole PEG 4000 was added to reaction mixture and the mixture was continuously stirred for 24 hrs.

The precipitate of dicyclohexyl urea was removed by filtration and the product was precipitated by slow addition of anhydrous diethyl ether and recrystallized with mixture of ether and dichloromethane (9:1). The yield was 2.9g and melting point was 45-46°C.

3.3.2 Preparation of Cloxacillin-conjugated PEG-dendrimer (C-3)

PEGylated cloxacillin 1.76 g (0.4 mmole) was dissolved in 40 ml of THF. To this solution 80.6 mg (0.4 mmole) of para-nitrophenylchloroformate (NPC) and 56 μl (0.4 mmole) triethylamine was added. The mixture was stirred for 24 hours at room temperature. The salt of triethylamine hydrochloride was filtered off. The filtrate was concentrated and drop wise added to diethyl ether. The precipitate was purified by reprecipitation from THF into diethyl ether. PEG-p-nitrophenylchloroformate (C-2) was recovered by evaporation under reduced pressure and recrystallized with ether and dichloromethane (9:1). Yield was 990 mg and percent yield was 54.09%.

To a solution of 22.08 mg (8µmole) EDTA core PAMAM dendrimer in dichloromethane (10ml), 160 µmole (736 mg) PEG-p-nitrophenylchloroformate was added and the solution was stirred for 72 h at room temperature. The reaction system was evaporated to dryness using rotary evaporation. The unreacted PEG and low molecular weight reagents were removed via ultra filtration. The product was recrystallized with ether and dichloromethane (9:1). Yield was 700 mg and percent yield was 91.68%. Melting point of derivatized cloxacillin was found at 52°C.

3.4 SYNTHESIS OF CEPHALEXIN-CONJUGATED PEG-DENDRIMER (D-3)

3.4.1 Synthesis of cephalexin conjugated PEG 4000 (D-1) via ester bond:

The synthesis was carried out following a general procedure given by Zalipsky et al[9](Scheme 2). 1.2 mmole (438 mg) of cephalexin was dissolved in 50 ml of dichloromethane and cooled in ice bath to 0°C. Then 1.3 mmole (268.2g) of DCC was added to solution with stirring following 1.2 mmole (146.6g) of DMAP (4-dimethylaminopyridine). After this addition 2 mmole PEG 4000 was added to reaction mixture and continuously stirred for 24 hrs.

The precipitate of dicyclohexyl urea was removed by filtration and the product was precipitated by slow addition of anhydrous diethyl ether. The product was recrystallized with mixture of ether and dichloromethane (9:1). The yield was 4.15g and percent yield was 79.56%. Melting point was found at 50°C.

3.4.2 Preparation of Cephalexin-conjugated PEG-dendrimer (D-3)

PEGylated cephalexin 1.739 g (0.4 mmole) was dissolved in 40 ml of THF. To this solution 80.6 mg (0.4 mmole) of pera-nitrophenylchloroformate (NPC) and 56 µl (0.4 mmole) triethylamine was added. The mixture was stirred for 24 hours at room temperature. The salt of triethylamine hydrochloride was filtered off. The filtrate was concentrated and drop wise added to diethyl ether. The precipitate was purified by reprecipitation from THF into diethyl ether. PEG-p-nitrophenylchloroformate (D-2) was recovered by evaporation under reduced pressure and recrystallized with ether and dichloromethane (9:1). Yield was 900 mg and percent yield was 49.47%.

To a solution of 22.08 mg (8μmole) EDTA core PAMAM dendrimer in dichloromethane (10ml), 160 μmole (736 mg) PEG-p-nitrophenylchloroformate was added and the solution was stirred for 72 h at room temperature. The reaction mixture was evaporated to dryness using rotary evaporation. The unreacted PEG and low molecular weight reagents were removed via ultra filtration. The product was recrystallized with ether and dichloromethane (9:1). Yield was 400 mg and percent yield was 64.23%. Melting point of derivatized cephalexin was found at 55°C.

3.5 SYNTHESIS OF CIPROFLOXACIN-CONJUGATED PEG-DENDRIMER (E3)

3.5.1 Synthesis of ciprofloxacin conjugated PEG 4000 (E-1) via ester bond:

The synthesis was done following a general procedure given by Zalipsky et al[9] (Scheme 2). 1.2 mmole (400 mg) of ciprofloxacin was dissolved in 50 ml of dichloromethane and cooled in ice bath to 0°C. Then 1.3 mmole (268.2g) of DCC was added to solution with stirring followed by 1.2 mmole (146.6g) of DMAP (4-dimethylaminopyridine) was added to the reaction mixture. After this addition 2 mmole PEG 4000 was added to reaction mixture and the mixture was continuously stirred for 24 hrs.

The precipitate of dicyclohexyl urea was removed by filtration and the product was precipitated by slow addition of anhydrous diethyl ether. The product was recrystallized with mixture of ether and dichloromethane (9:1). The yield was 3.3g and percent yield was 63.49%. Melting point was found at 50-52°C.

3.5.2 Preparation of Ciprofloxacin-conjugated PEG-dendrimer (E-3)

PEGylated ciprofloxacin 1.725 g (0.4 mmole) was dissolved in 40 ml of THF. To this solution 80.6 mg (0.4 mmole) of pera-nitrophenylchloroformate (NPC) and 56 μl (0.4 mmole) triethylamine were added and stirred for 24 hours at room temperature. The salt of triethylamine hydrochloride was filtered off. The filtrate was concentrated and dropwise added to diethyl ether. The precipitate was purified by reprecipitation from THF into diethyl ether. PEG-p-nitrophenylchloroformate (E-2) was recovered by evaporation under reduced pressure and recrystallized with ether and dichloromethane (9:1). Yield was 1.05g and percent yield was 58.33%.

To a solution of 22.08 mg (8μmole) EDTA core PAMAM dendrimer in dichloromethane (10ml), 160 μmole (600 mg) PEG-p-nitrophenylchloroformate was added and the solution was stirred for 72 hrs. at room temperature. The reaction system was evaporated to dryness using rotary evaporation. The unreacted PEG and low molecular weight reagents were removed via ultra filtration. The product was recrystallized with ether and dichloromethane (9:1). Yield was 610 mg and percent yield was 97.92%. Melting point of derivatized ciprofloxacin was found at 50-52°C.

CHARACTERIZATION OF SYNTHESIZED PRODUCTS

For characterizing intermediates and final products, normal course of characterization, *viz.*, spectroscopic methods are used along with physicochemical constants like melting point, elemental composition *etc.*

Characterization of Intermediates and drug derivatized complexes

Solubility:

Solubility can be defined quantitatively as the concentration of the solute in a saturated solution at a certain temperature; I. P. (1996) expresses solubility at the temperature ranging from 20° – 30° C.

Procedure:

Approximately 10mg of compound was dissolved in 5 mL of each solvent at 37± 1° C in glass test tubes. Test tubes were gently shaken and solubilities were observed. In case of any observed insoluble fraction, the known amount of solvent was further added to ascertain the solubility of the product. The solubility of various synthesized product was studied in various solvents. The observations are recorded in Table 3.1.

Determination of Melting Point:

The melting points of the synthesized intermediates and derivatized drugs were determined by open capillary tube using Mvtex melting point apparatus and are uncorrected. The melting points are recorded in Table 3.1.

Table 3.1: Solubility data of Intermediates and derivatized drugs

S.NO.	Comp. Code	Water	Ethanol	Methanol	Chloroform	DCM	Benzene
1.	G1.0	+	+++	+++	+	-	-
2.	G1.5	+++	++	+	+	-	-
3.	G2.0	-	+	+	+++	++	-
4.	G2.5	-	+	+	+++	++	-
5.	G3.0	-	+	+	+++	++	-
6.	C-1	-	+	+	+++	++	-
7.	C-2	-	+	+	+++	++	-
8.	C-3	-	+	+	+++	++	-
9.	D-1	-	+	+	+++	++	-
10.	D-2	-	+	+	+++	++	-
11.	D-3	-	+	+	+++	++	-
12.	E-1	-	+	+	+++	++	-
13.	E-2	-	+	+	+++	++	-
14.	E-3	-	+	+	+++	++	-

Solubility Denotations: - Insoluble, +Slightly soluble, ++ Moderately soluble, +++ Highly soluble

Table 3.2 Physicochemical data of synthesized compounds

S.NO.	Comp. Code	Melting Point	Recrystallization Solvent	Percent Yield	%Nitrogen Calculated	%Nitrogen Found
1.	G1.0	140°C	Water & Ethanol	95.33%	30.14	29.98
2.	G1.5	199°D	Water & Ethanol	31.66%	15.14	14.96
3.	G2.0	190°C	Water & Ethanol	78.18%	28.87	27.90
4.	G2.5	200°C	Water & Ethanol	38.80%	16.20	16.05
5.	G3.0	145°C	Water & Ethanol	96.15%	28.17	27.99
6.	C-3	52°C	Ether & DCM	91.68%	1.96	1.89
7.	D-3	55°C	Ether & DCM	64.23%	1.98	1.93
8.	E-3	50°C	Ether & DCM	96.32%	1.98	1.95

Elemental Analysis (Nitrogen): Elemental analysis of synthesized compounds was done by elemental analyzer (Vario EL-III) for nitrogen. The percentage nitrogen content found and calculated were almost similar for the synthesized compounds as shown in Table 3.2.

Infrared Spectroscopy:

The IR spectra of the products were recorded on FTIR spectrophotometer (Schimadzu 8400S) in KBr pellets. The principal peaks shown in the spectra along with their wave number are shown in table no. 3.3-3.5, 3.7-3.8, 3.10, 3.12, 3.14, 3.16, 3.18, 3.20 and 3.22.

H^1 NMR Spectroscopy:

The PMR spectral analyses of the synthesized products were done on NMR spectrophotometer (Bruker DRX 300) using Deutearated DMSO as solvent. The peaks shown in the spectra along with their interpretation are recorded and shown in table no. 3.6, 3.9, 3.11, 3.13, 3.15, 3.17, 3.19, 3.21 and 3.23. The spectral data obtained was interpreted with help of appropriate spectral correlation chart[10].

Structure of compound G 0 (starting material for dendrimer synthesis)

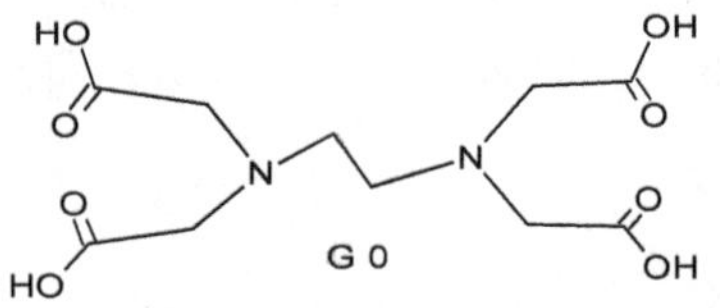

(E.D.T.A.)

FTIR spectrum of E.D.T.A. (G 0)

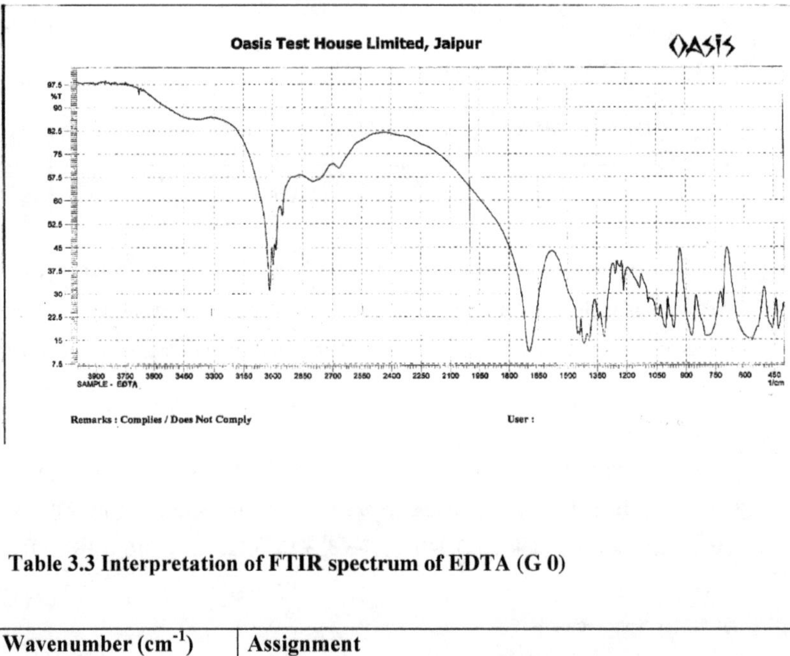

Table 3.3 Interpretation of FTIR spectrum of EDTA (G 0)

Wavenumber (cm^{-1})	Assignment
3300-2550	The O-H stretching absorption of carboxylic acid dimer
2997-2950	Aliphatic C-H stretching
1697	The C=O stretching of carboxylic dimer

Structure of compound G 1.0

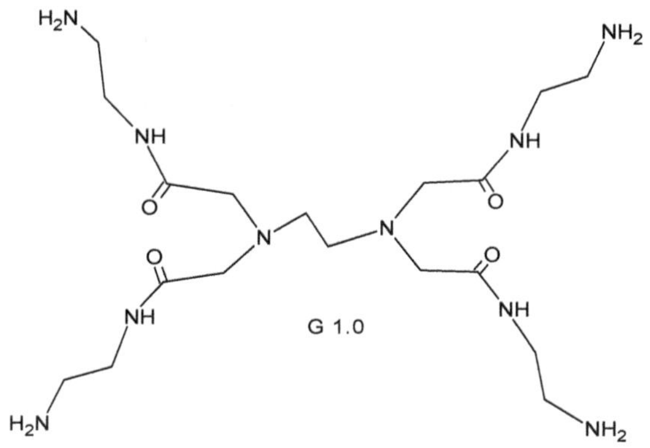

FTIR spectrum of compound G 1.0

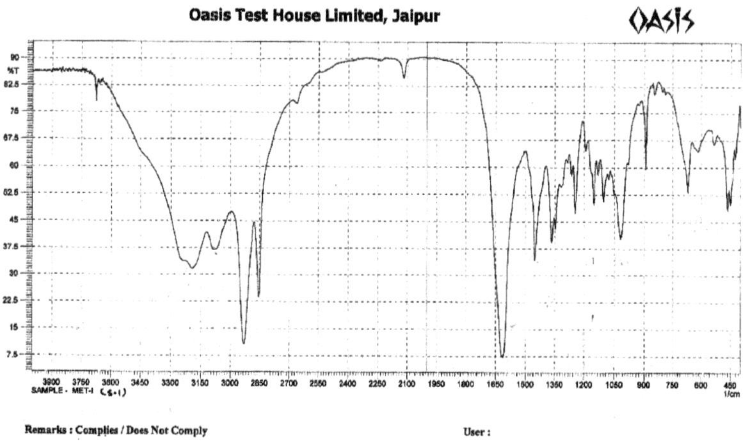

Table 3.4 Interpretation of FTIR spectrum of EDTA (G 1.0)

Wave number (cm^{-1})	Assignment
3244	The N-H stretch of secondary amine
3191 & 3083	Asymmetric and symmetric N-H stretch, hydrogen bonded, primary amine coupled doublet
2929 & 2854	Aliphatic asymmetric and symmetric C-H stretching
1614	The C=O stretching of amide
1452	The C-N stretch
700-600	The broad N-H out of plane band of primary amine

Structure of compound G 1.5

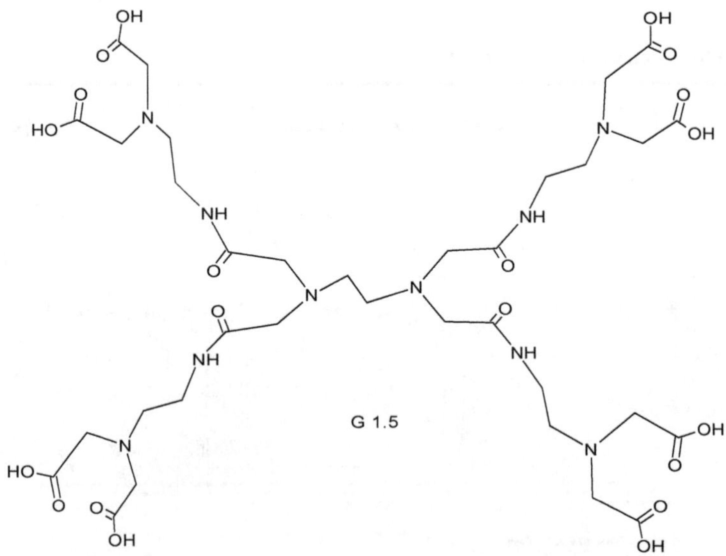

G 1.5

FTIR spectrum of compound G 1.5

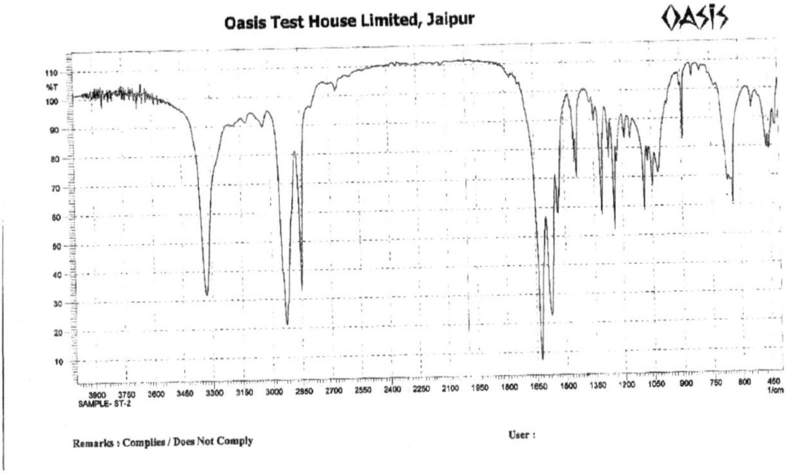

Table 3.5 Interpretation of FTIR spectrum of E.D.T.A. (G 1.5)

Wave number (cm^{-1})	Assignment
3326	The N-H stretch of secondary amine (singlet)
2927 & 2850	Aliphatic asymmetric and symmetric C-H stretching
1626	The C=O stretching of acid
1574	The C=O stretch of amide
1436	The C-O-H in plane band
1244	The C-O stretch

H^1-NMR spectrum of G1.5 compound

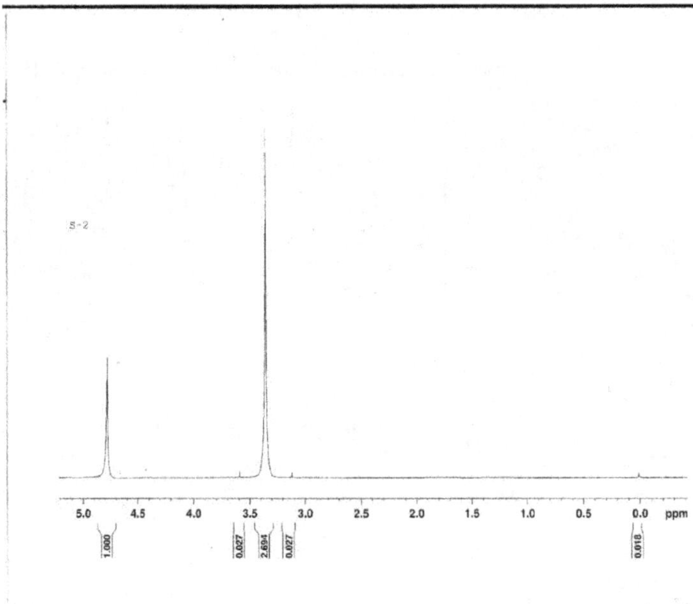

Table 3.6 Interpretation of H^1-NMR spectrum of G1.5 compound

Observed Value (δ ppm)	Signal due to
3.359	Due to $-CH_2$ protons of ethylenediamine parts of the compound
4.785	Due to $-CH_2$ protons present in between carbonyl and tertiary amino groups of compound

Structure of compound G 2.0

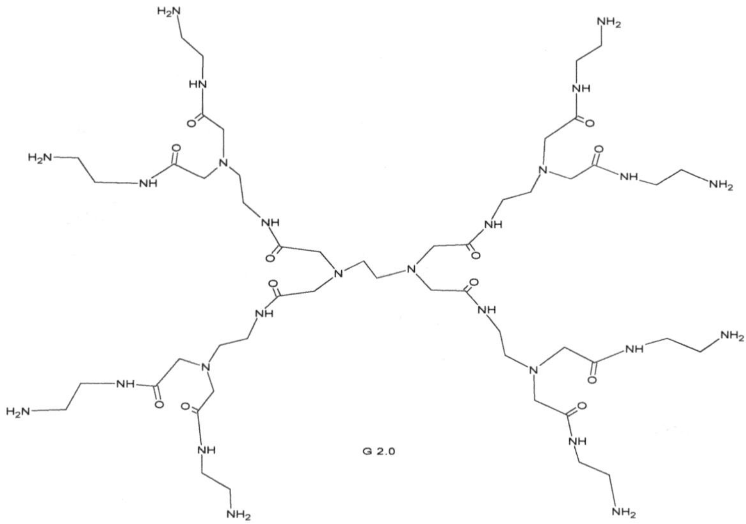

FTIR spectrum of compound G 2.0

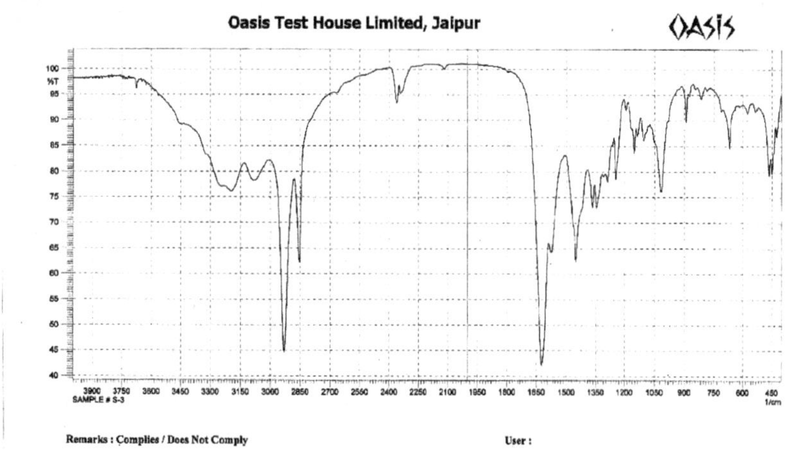

Table 3.7 Interpretation of FTIR spectrum of compound G 2.0

Wave number (cm^{-1})	Assignment
3244	The N-H stretch of secondary amine
3195 & 3082	Asymmetric and symmetric N-H stretch, hydrogen bonded, primary amine coupled doublet
2929 & 2854	Aliphatic asymmetric and symmetric C-H stretching
1623	The C=O stretching of amide
1452	The C-N stretch

Structure of compound G 2.5

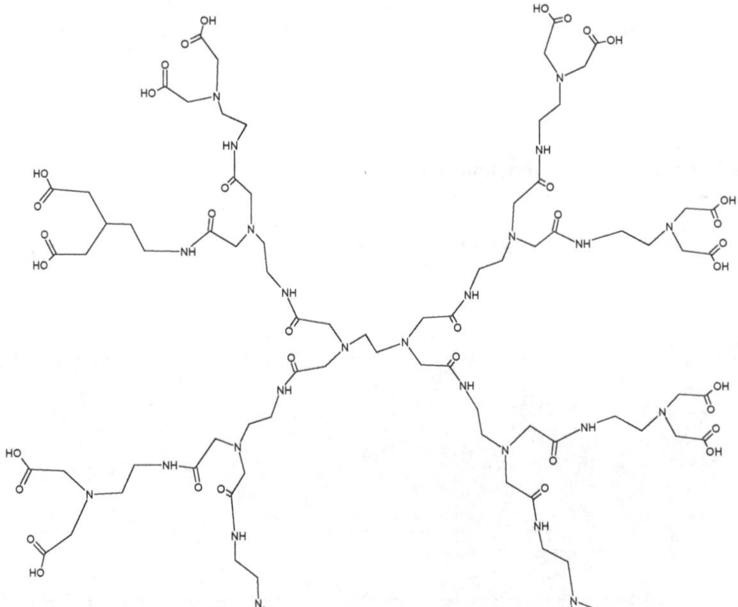

G 2.5

FTIR spectrum of compound G 2.5

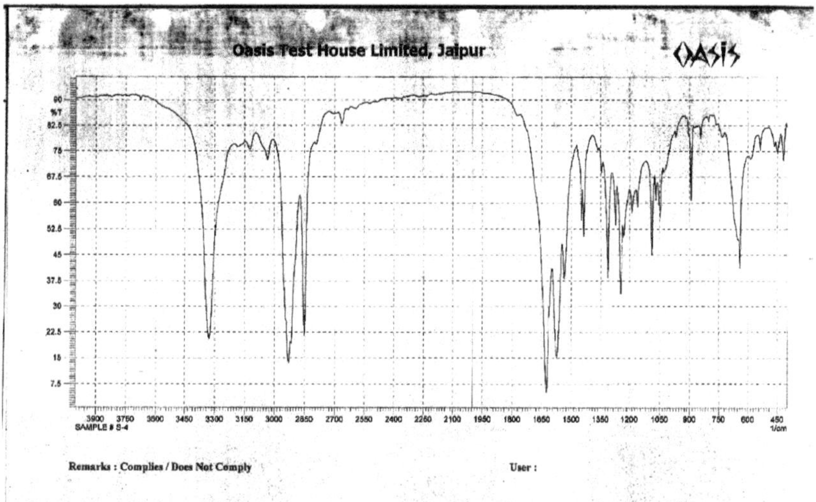

Table 3.8 Interpretation of FTIR spectra of compound G 2.5

Wave number (cm^{-1})	Assignment
3327	The N-H stretch of secondary amine (singlet)
2928 & 2850	Aliphatic asymmetric and symmetric C-H stretching
1626	The C=O stretching of acid
1574	The C=O stretch of amide
1436	The C-O-H in plane bend

H^1-NMR spectrum of compound G 2.5

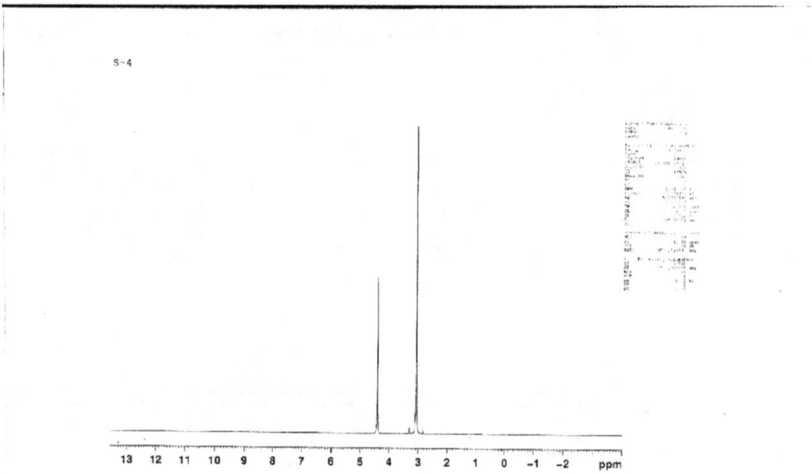

Table 3.9 Interpretation of H^1-NMR spectrum of compound G 2.5

Observed Value (δ ppm)	Signal due to
3.08	Due to $-CH_2$ protons of ethylenediamino parts of the compound
4.30	Due to $-CH_2$ protons present in between carbonyl and tertiary amino groups of compound

Structure of compound G 3.0 (Final Dendrimer)

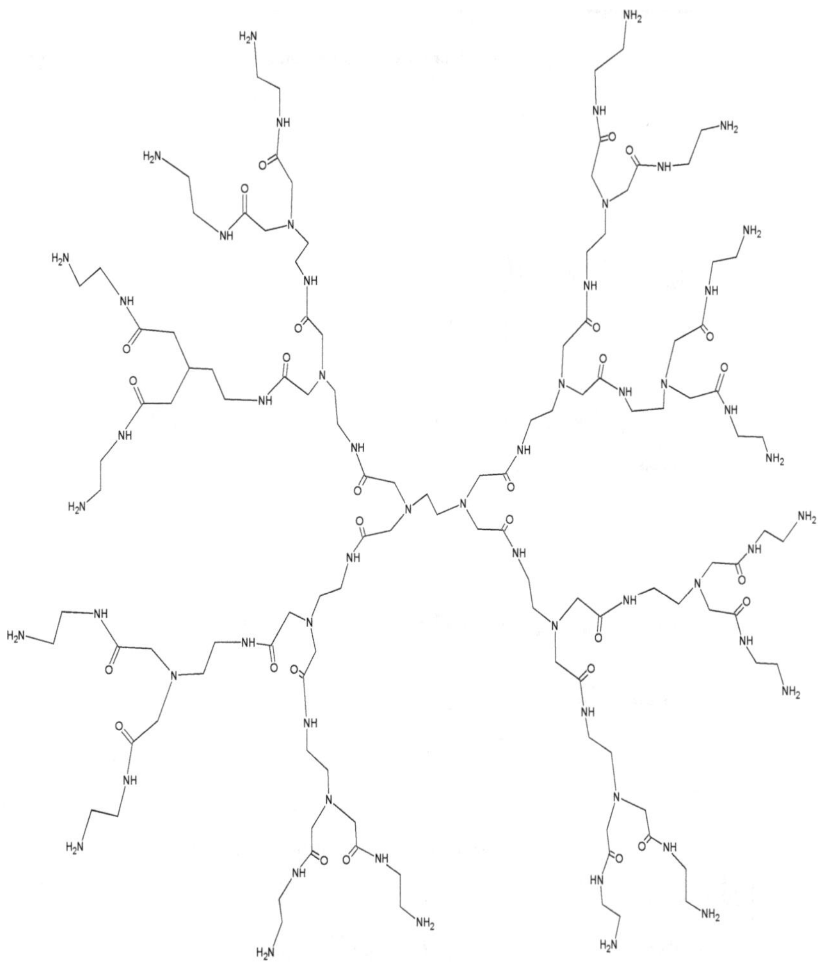

G 3.0

FTIR spectrum of compound G 3.0

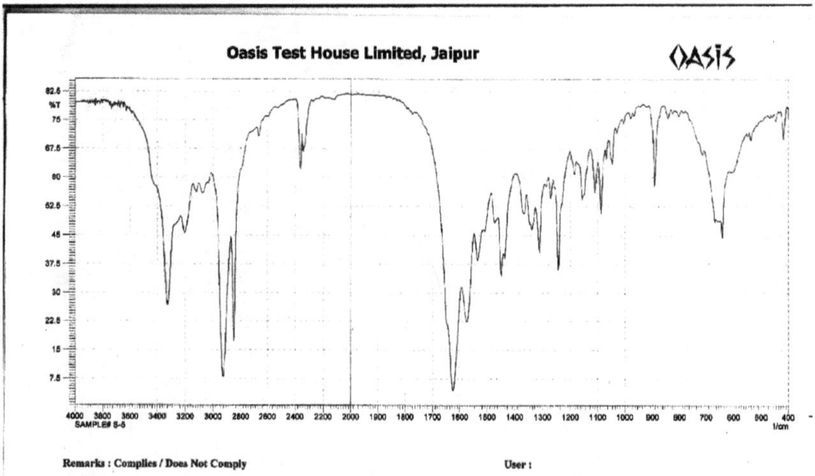

Table 3.10 Interpretation of FTIR spectrum of compound G 3.0

Wave number (cm^{-1})	Assignment
3327	The N-H stretch of secondary amine (singlet)
3205 & 3124	Asymmetric and symmetric N-H stretch of hydrogen bonded primary amine (coupled doublet)
2929 & 2854	Aliphatic asymmetric and symmetric C-H stretching
1626-1535	The C=O stretch of amides

H^1-NMR spectrum of compound G 3.0

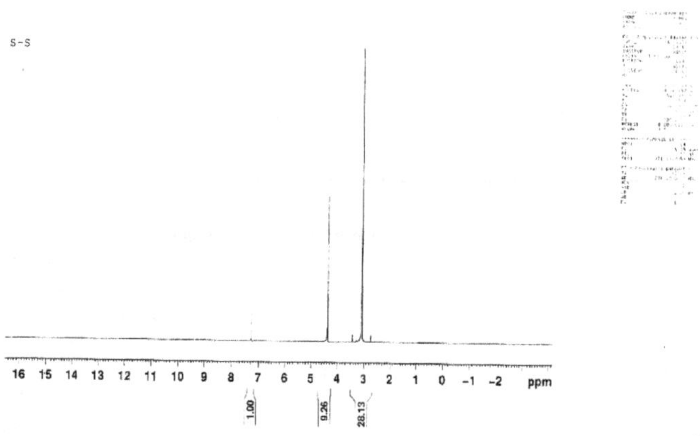

Table 3.11 Interpretation of H^1-NMR spectrum of compound G 3.0

Observed Value (δ ppm)	Signal due to
3.10	Due to $-CH_2$ protons of ethylenediamine parts of the compound
4.50	Due to $-CH_2$ protons present in between carbonyl and tertiary amine groups of compound
7.26	Due to protons attached to nitrogen atom in compound

Structure of Cloxacillin conjugated PEG 4000

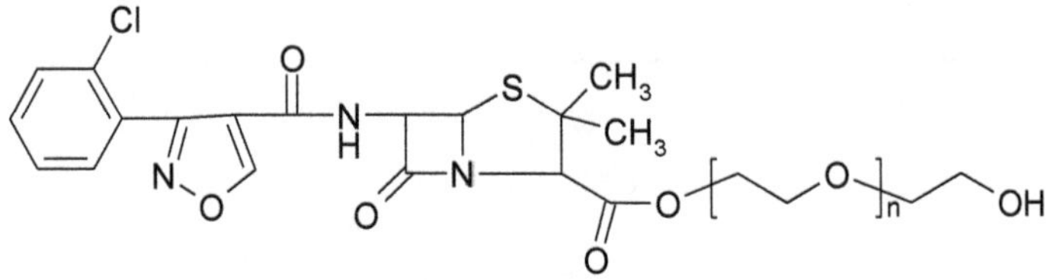

FTIR spectrum of Cloxacillin conjugated PEG 4000

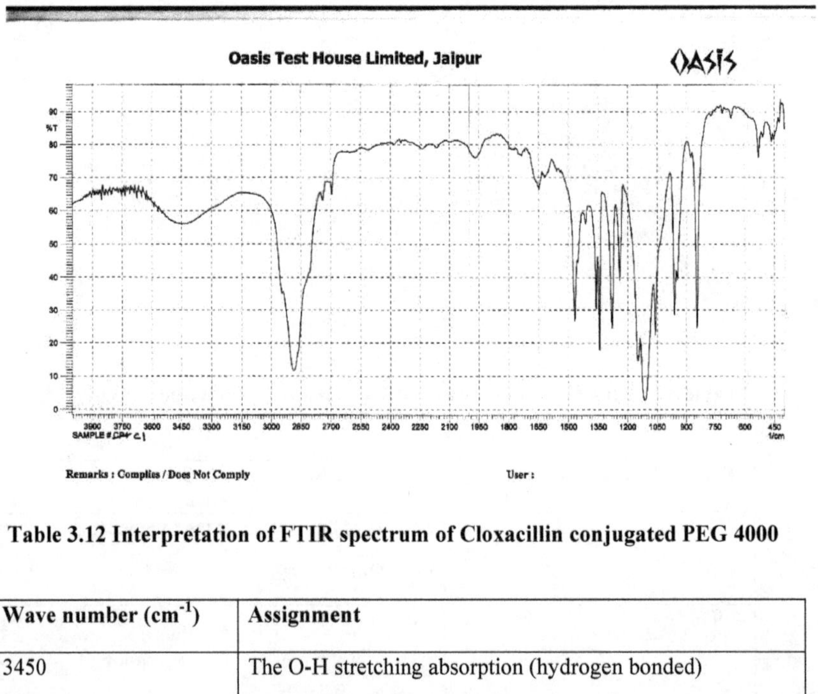

Table 3.12 Interpretation of FTIR spectrum of Cloxacillin conjugated PEG 4000

Wave number (cm^{-1})	Assignment
3450	The O-H stretching absorption (hydrogen bonded)
2945 & 2885	Aliphatic asymmetric and symmetric C-H stretching
1650	The C=O stretching of cloxacillin
1150 & 1170	The C-O-C stretching of polyethylene glycol

H^1-NMR of Cloxacillin conjugated PEG 4000

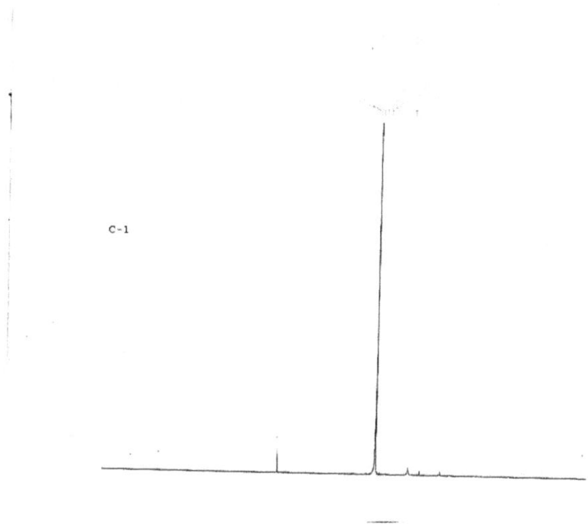

Table 3.13 Interpretation of H^1-NMR spectrum of Cloxacillin conjugated PEG 4000

Observed Value (δ ppm)	Signal due to
1.25	Due to $-CH_3$ protons of cloxacillin
3.64	Due to protons of PEG 4000 $-(O-CH_2-CH_2)-$
7.25-7.27	Due to protons of $-C_6H_5$ in cloxacillin

Structure of Cloxacillin-conjugated PEG-dendrimer

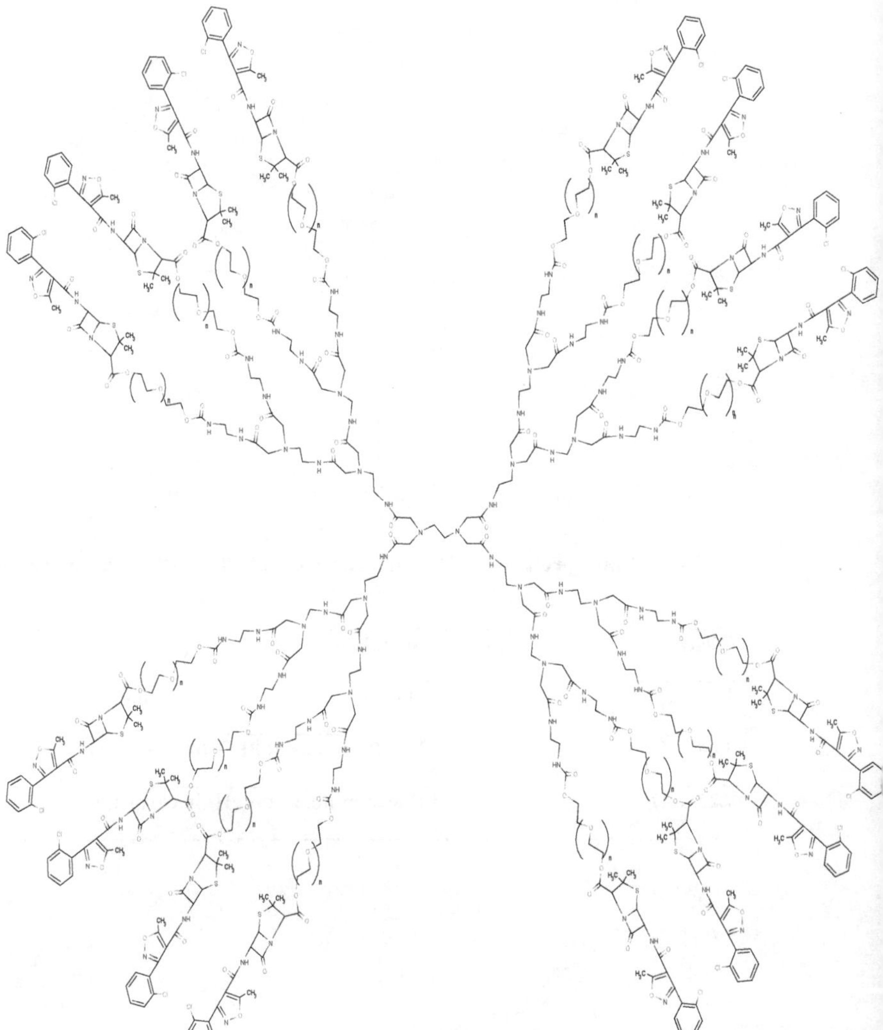

FTIR spectrum of Cloxacillin-conjugated PEG-dendrimer

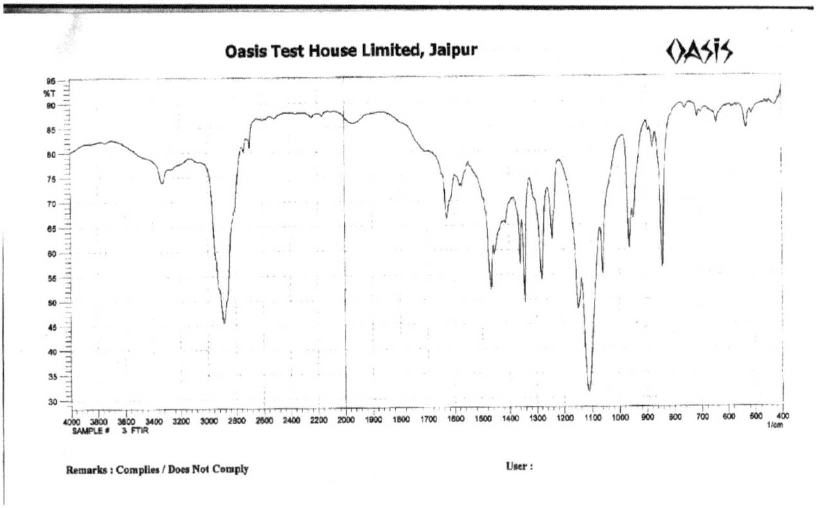

Table 3.14 Interpretation of FTIR spectrum of Cloxacillin-conjugated PEG-dendrimer

Wavelength (cm^{-1})	Assignment
3427	The N-H stretch of dendrimer (singlet)
2991	Aliphatic C-H stretching
1656	The C=O stretching
1466	The C-N stretch
1109 & 1140	The C-O-C stretch

H^1-NMR spectrum of Cloxacillin-conjugated PEG-dendrimer

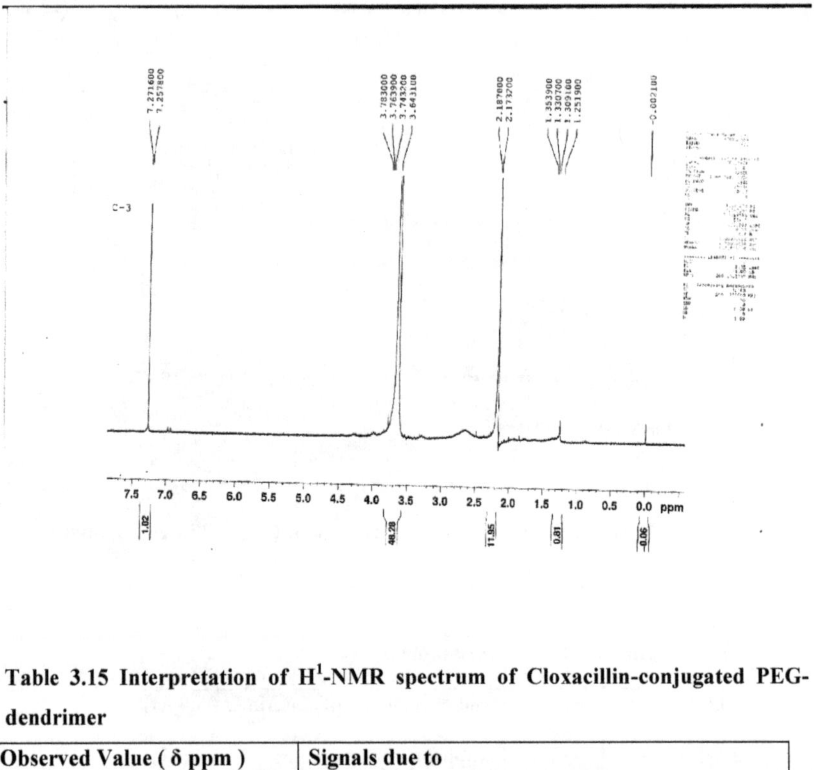

Table 3.15 Interpretation of H^1-NMR spectrum of Cloxacillin-conjugated PEG-dendrimer

Observed Value (δ ppm)	Signals due to
1.25-1.35	Due to $-CH_3$ protons of cloxacillin
2.17-2.18	Due to protons of dendrimer
3.64-3.78	Due to protons of PEG 4000 $-(O-CH_2-CH_2)-$
7.25-7.27	Due to protons of $-C_6H_5$ in cloxacillin

Structure of Cephalexin conjugated PEG 4000

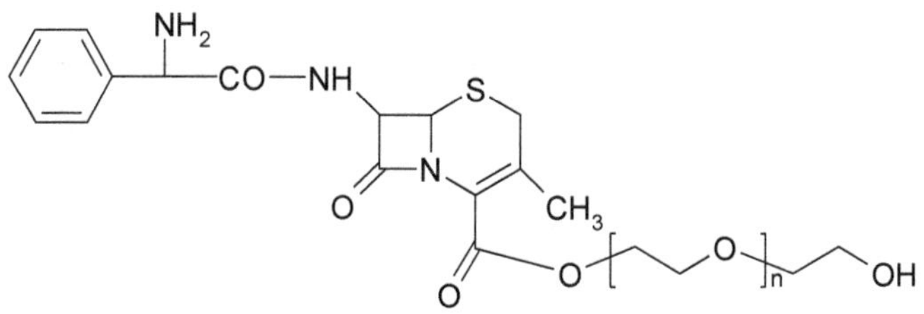

FTIR spectrum of Cephalexin conjugated PEG 4000

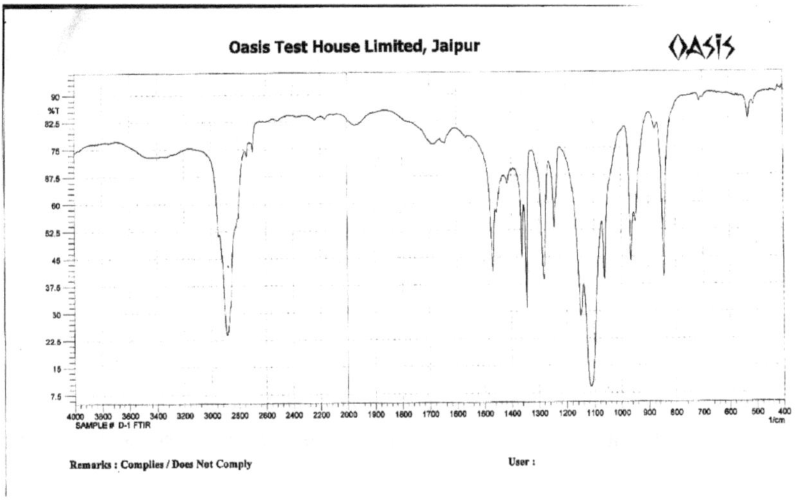

Table 3.16 Interpretation of FTIR spectrum of Cephalexin conjugated PEG 4000

Wavelength (cm^{-1})	Assignment
3400	The O-H stretching absorption (hydrogen bonded)
2945 & 2885	Aliphatic asymmetric and symmetric C-H stretching
1650	The C=O stretching of cephalexin
1150	The C-O-C stretching of polyethylene glycol

H^1-NMR spectrum of Cephalexin conjugated PEG 4000

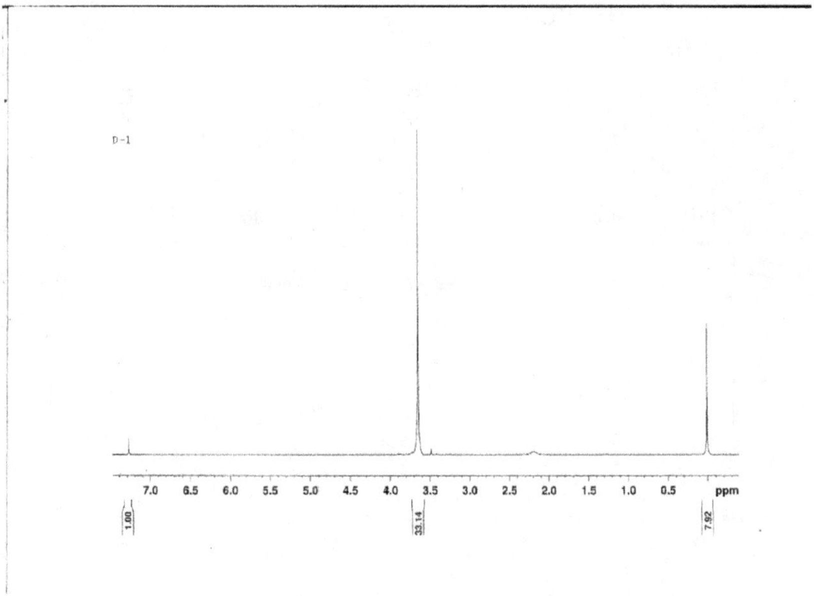

Table 3.17 Interpretation of H^1-NMR spectrum of Cephalexin conjugated PEG 4000

Observed Value (δ ppm)	Signal due to
1.26-1.29	Due to –CH_3 protons of cephalexin
3.60-3.73	Due to protons of PEG 4000 –(O-CH_2-CH_2)-
7.28-7.33	Due to protons of -C_6H_5 in cephalexin

Structure of Cephalexin-conjugated PEG-dendrimer

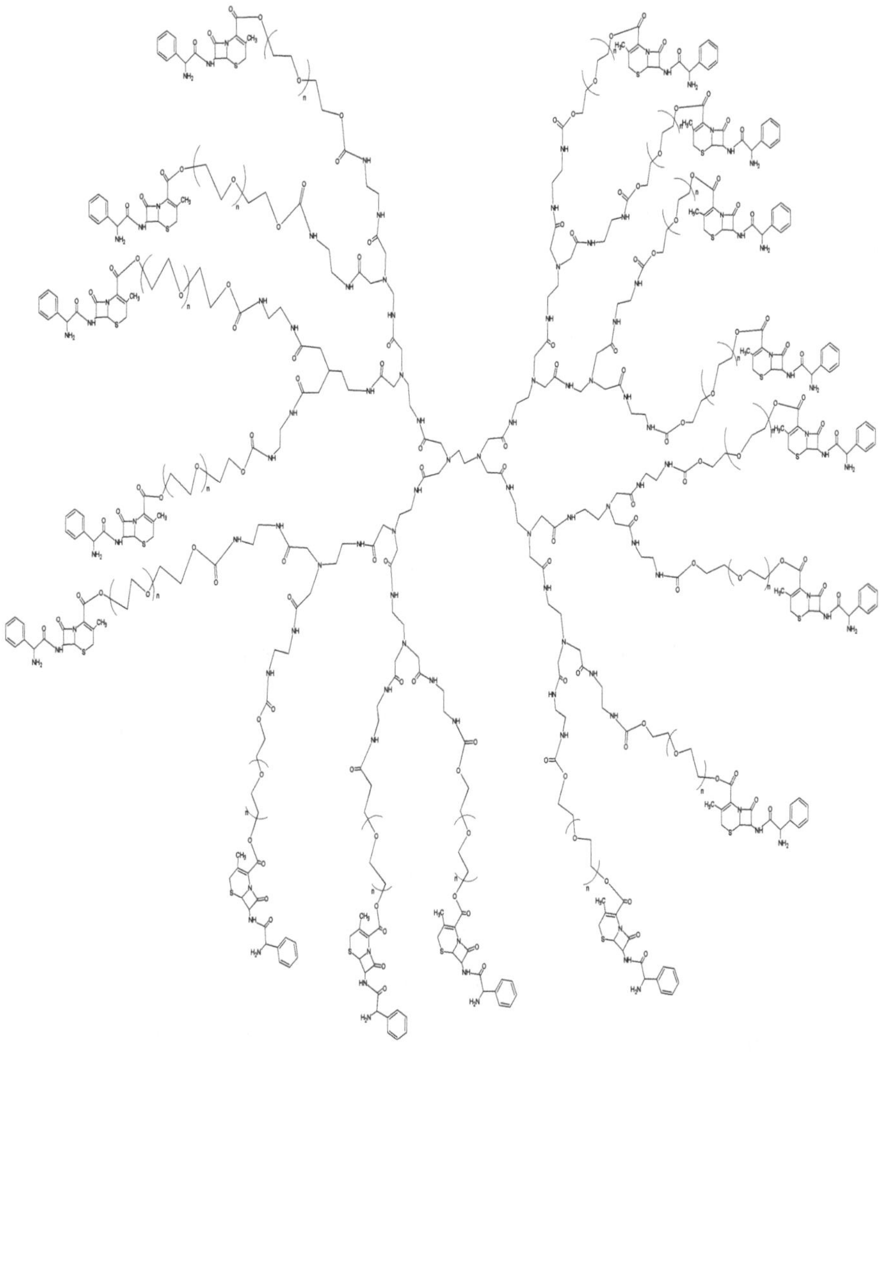

FTIR spectrum of Cephalexin-conjugated PEG-dendrimer

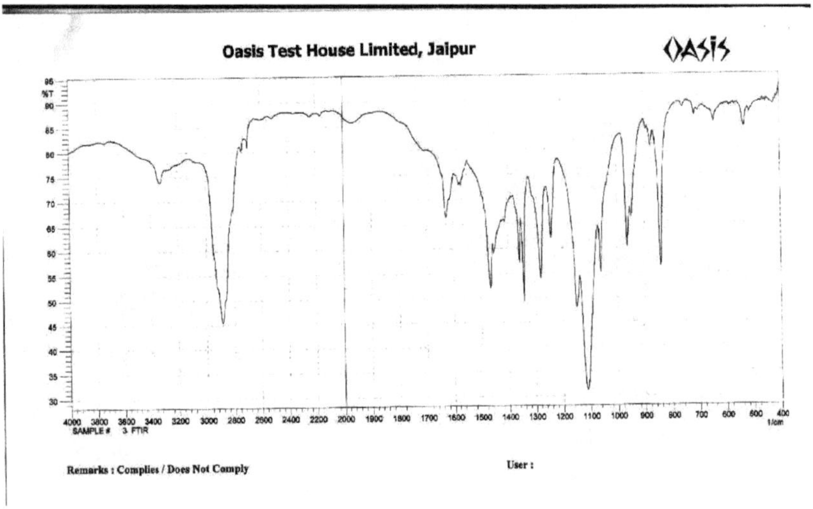

Table 3.18 Interpretation of FTIR spectrum of Cephalexin-conjugated PEG-dendrimer

Wavelength (cm^{-1})	Assignment
3320	The N-H stretch of secondary amine of dendrimer (singlet)
2887 & 2806	Aliphatic asymmetric and symmetric C-H stretching
1627	The C=O stretching of dendrimer (C=O stretching of cephalexin is merged in it)
1467	The C-N stretch
1110 & 1140	The C-O-C stretch of polyethylene glycol

H^1-NMR spectrum of Cephalexin-conjugated PEG-dendrimer

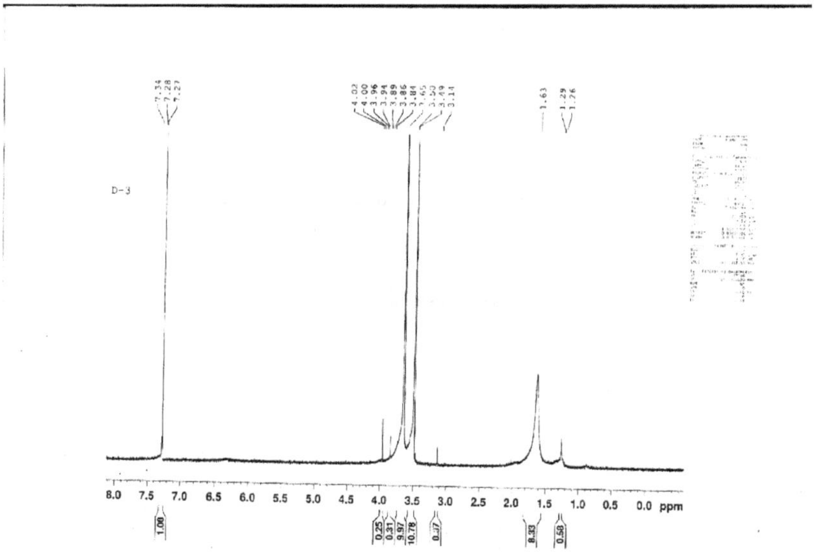

Table 3.19 Interpretation of H^1-NMR spectrum of Cephalexin-conjugated PEG-dendrimer

Observed Value (δ ppm)	Signal due to
1.26-1.29	Due to $-CH_3$ protons of cephalexin
1.63	Due to protons of dendrimer
3.49-3.65	Due to protons of PEG 4000 $-(O-CH_2-CH_2)-$
7.27-7.34	Due to protons of $-C_6H_5$ in cephalexin

Structure of Ciprofloxacin conjugated PEG 4000

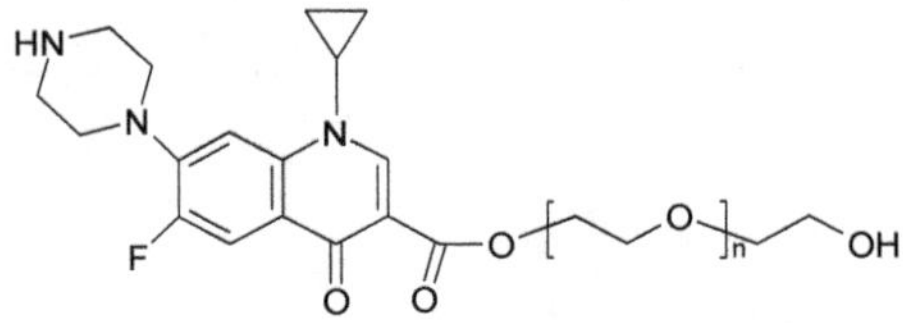

FTIR spectrum of Ciprofloxacin conjugated PEG 4000

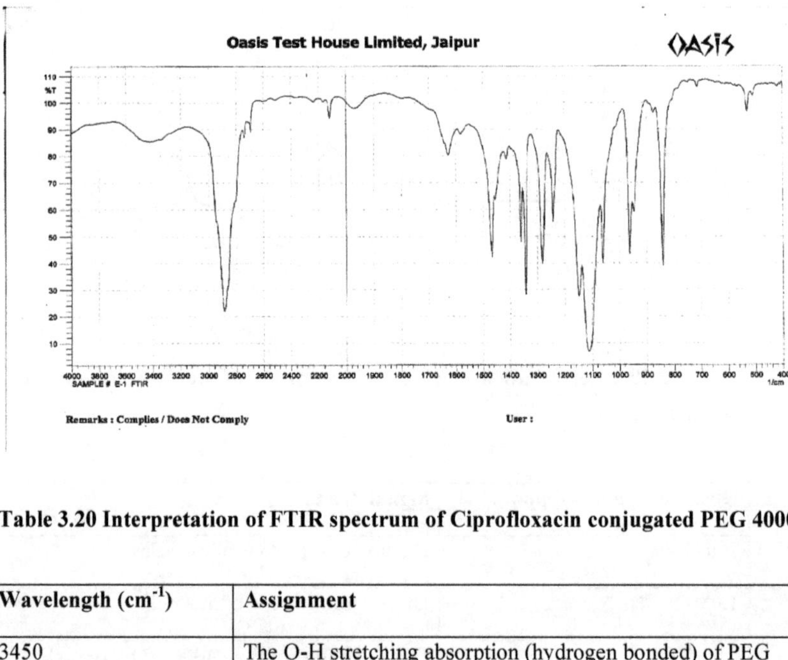

Table 3.20 Interpretation of FTIR spectrum of Ciprofloxacin conjugated PEG 4000

Wavelength (cm^{-1})	Assignment
3450	The O-H stretching absorption (hydrogen bonded) of PEG
2885 & 2806	Aliphatic asymmetric and symmetric C-H stretching
1640	The C=O stretching of ciprofloxacin
1110	The C-O-C stretching of polyethylene glycol

H[1]-NMR spectrum of Ciprofloxacin conjugated PEG 4000

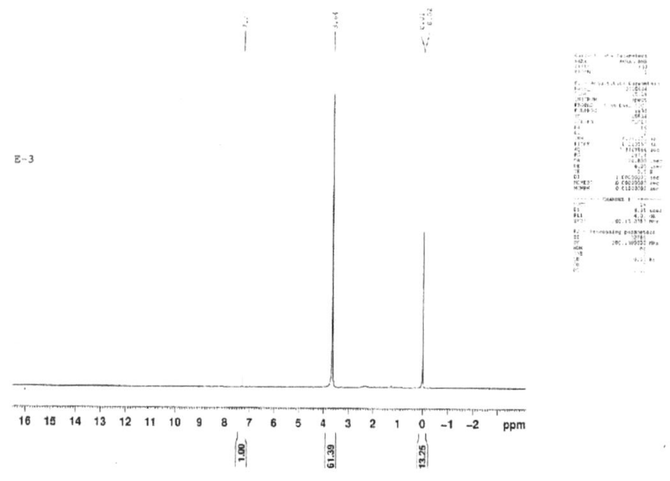

Table 3.21 Interpretation of H[1]-NMR spectrum of Ciprofloxacin conjugated PEG 4000

Observed Value (δ ppm)	Signal due to
1.25-1.36	Due to $-CH_2$ protons of ciprofloxacin
3.64	Due to protons of PEG 4000 $-(O-CH_2-CH_2)-$
7.27	Due to protons of phenyl ring in ciprofloxacin

Structure of Ciprofloxacin-conjugated PEG-dendrimer

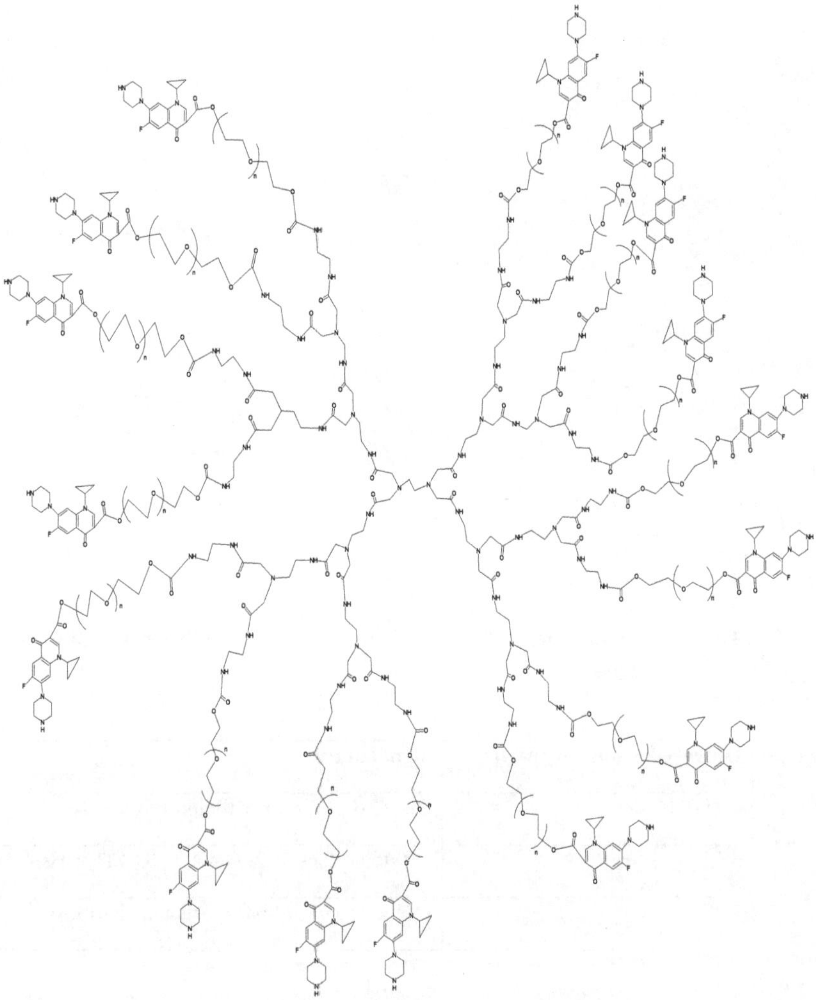

FTIR spectrum of Ciprofloxacin-conjugated PEG-dendrimer

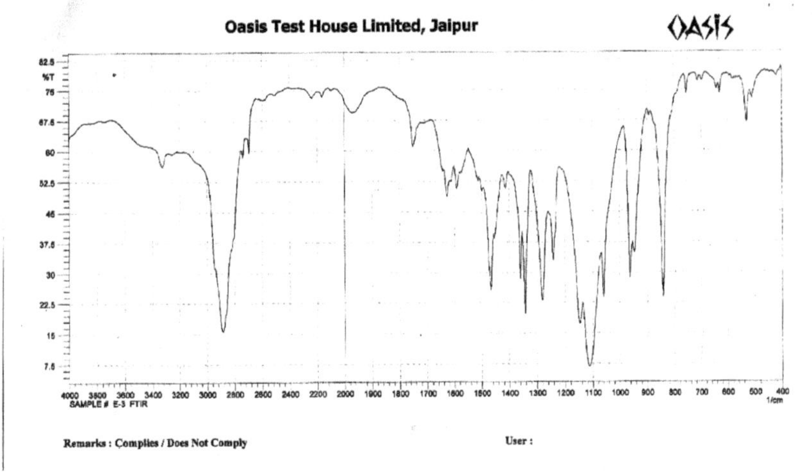

Table 3.22 Interpretation of FTIR spectrum of Ciprofloxacin-conjugated PEG-dendrimer

Wavelength (cm^{-1})	Assignment
3320	The N-H stretch of secondary amine of dendrimer (singlet)
2887 & 2806	Aliphatic asymmetric and symmetric C-H stretching
1751	The C=O stretching of ciprofloxacin
1627	The C=O stretching of dendrimer
1109 & 1140	The C-O-C stretching of PEG (symmetric and asymmetric)

H[1]-NMR spectrum of Ciprofloxacin-conjugated PEG-dendrimer

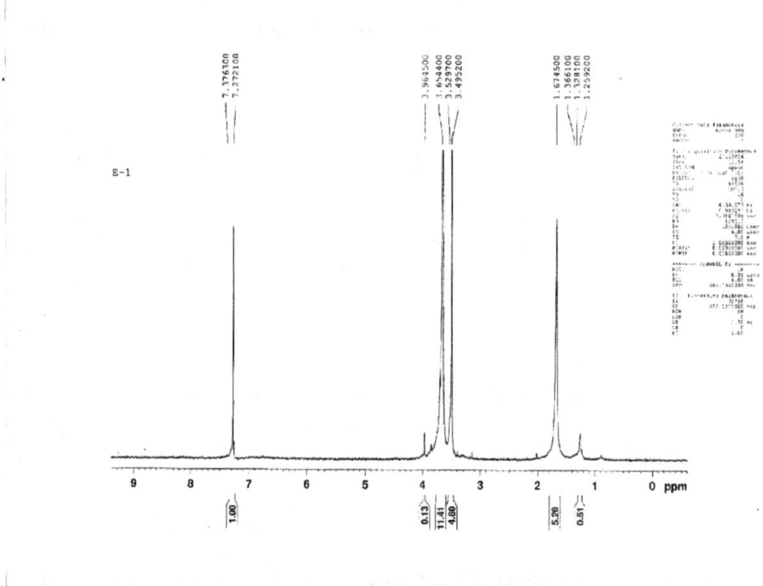

Table 3.23 Interpretation of H[1]-NMR spectrum of Ciprofloxacin-conjugated PEG-dendrimer

Observed Value (δ ppm)	Signal due to
1.25-1.36	Due to $-CH_2$ protons of ciprofloxacin
1.67	Due to protons of dendrimer
3.49-3.65	Due to protons of PEG 4000 $-(O-CH_2-CH_2)-$
7.27-7.37	Due to protons of phenyl ring in ciprofloxacin

RESULT AND DISCUSSION

The synthesis of novel EDTA core PAMAM Dendrimer was executed in five linear steps from EDTA as a starting material with 68% overall yield. Divergent method of synthesis was used in which EDTA was reacted with ethylene diamine in the presence of DCC and the obtained amine was reacted with formaldehyde, sodium cyanide and water to form acid functional group. These two reaction steps were repeated to form final G 3.0 PAMAM dendrimer. Synthesis of drug derivatives was also done satisfactorily. EDTA core PAMAM Dendrimer was aimed to synthesize drug derivatives of the drugs bearing carboxylic or sulphonic groups.

Drug derivatives of cloxacillin, cephalexin and ciprofloxacin using PEG-4000 as spacer groups were synthesized in three steps (Scheme 2). First step was synthesis of drug conjugated PEG 4000 via ester bond. This was done by reacting drug with PEG in the presence of DCC and DMAP. Using terminal hydroxyl groups of PEG to couple with carboxylic group containing drug is straightforward way for esterification. In order to obtain a high percentage of mono-functionalized PEG, a large reaction volume, high ratio of free PEG to selected carboxylic group containing drugs and low temperature were employed. In second step PEGylated drug was activated by para nitrophenylchloroformate into the active carbonate form which readily reacts with dendrimer surface primary amino groups.

In third step EDTA core PAMAM dendrimers having 16 free $-NH_2$ groups were reacted with PEGylated drug intermediate to form final drug derivatives. In our study the mole ratio of PEG to dendrimer core was over 1.0 to make sure that surface of dendrimer was saturated with PEG arms. These intermediates and final drug derivatives were characterized by spectroscopic methods along with physicochemical parameters like melting point, element composition *etc.* Their solubility data are recorded in Table 3.1. It reveals that these intermediates are more lipophilic and their solubility is less in water as compared to drugs and spacer moieties. Their physical description, melting point, element composition are reported in Table 3.2. Characteristic absorption peaks obtained in FTIR and PMR spectra along with interpretation are reported in Table 3.3 to 3.23.

Initially the intermediates were characterized. Their nitrogen content was near to calculated nitrogen content as shown in table 3.2. Their spectroscopic characterizations were done by FTIR and proton NMR analysis.

The FTIR spectrum of pure EDTA gave broad band at 3300-2550 cm^{-1}, showing the presence of O-H stretching absorption of carboxylic acid dimer and a band at 1697 cm^{-1}, showing the carbonyl stretching of carboxylic dimer.

After reacting with ethylenediamine free carboxylic group of EDTA was converted into amide bond having four free amino groups on surface (G 1.0). Now compound G 1.0 have three types of nitrogen 1°, 2° and 3° in their structures and these types of nitrogen were confirmed by FTIR of G 1.0. Absorption band at 3244 cm^{-1} showed the N-H stretch of secondary amine and a doublet at 3191 & 3083 showed the asymmetric and symmetric stretch of N-H of primary amine of G 1.0.

Then G 1.0 was reacted with HCHO, NaCN and water, which replaced the hydrogens of free amine with $-CH_2COOH$ groups to form compound G 1.5. This was confirmed by disappearance of doublet of primary amino group and appearance of carbonyl stretching of carboxylic group at 1626 cm^{-1} in the FTIR spectrum of G 1.5. The two types of protons of G 1.5 were confirmed by proton NMR spectra showing two peaks at δ 3.359 and 4.785 ppm. Deshielding of methylene protons present in between nitrogen and carbonyl group was found higher (δ 4.785) than ethylene protons in between nitrogens (δ 3.359) as predictive.

Then the carboxylic groups of G 1.5 were converted into free primary amine groups by reacting with ethylene diamine and compound G 2.0 was obtained. This conversion was confirmed by the appearance of primary amino doublet at 3195 and 3082 cm^{-1} in FTIR spectrum of G 2.0.

The compound G 2.0 was reacted with HCHO, NaCN and water, which replaced the hydrogens of free amine with $-CH_2COOH$ groups to form compound G 2.5. This was confirmed by disappearance of doublet of primary amino group and appearance of carbonyl stretching of carboxylic group at 1626 cm^{-1} in the FTIR spectrum of G 2.5. The two types of protons of G 2.5 were confirmed by proton NMR spectrum showing two peaks at δ 3.08 and 4.30 ppm. One type of protons is ethylene group which is present in between two nitrogens and another type is methylene which is present in between nitrogen and carbonyl groups.

Deshielding of methylene protons present in between nitrogen and carbonyl group was found higher (δ 4.30) than ethylene protons in between nitrogens (δ 3.08) as predictive.

Then the carboxylic group of G 2.5 was again converted into free primary amino groups by reacting with ethylene diamine and compound G 3.0 was obtained. This conversion was confirmed by the appearance of primary amino doublet at 3205 and 3124 cm^{-1} in FTIR spectrum of G 3.0. The three types of protons of compound G 3.0 were confirmed by proton NMR spectrum showing three signals at δ 3.10, 4.50 and 7.26 ppm. One type of protons is ethylene group which is present in between two nitrogens showing peak at 3.10 ppm and second type of proton is methylene which is present in between nitrogen and carbonyl groups showing peak at 4.50 ppm. Deshielding of methylene protons present in between nitrogen and carbonyl group was found higher (δ 4.50) than ethylene protons in between nitrogens (δ 3.10) as predictive. Third type of protons is of primary amino group which present on surface of final dendrimer (G 3.0) is showing peak at 7.26 ppm as predictive because they are directly attached to electronegative nitrogen atom producing higher amount of deshielding to protons.

Thus in the light of these evidences it can be concluded that the novel EDTA core dendrimer was synthesized satisfactorily.

Similarly the PEGylated cloxacillin, cephalexin and ciprofloxacin were also characterized.

The FTIR spectra of PEGylated cloxacillin, cephalexin and ciprofloxacin show some common bands of polyethylene glycol which is a bigger part of the conjugates. The O-H stretching absorption band (hydrogen bonded) at around 3450 cm^{-1} and aliphatic asymmetric & symmetric stretch appears at around 2850-2950 cm^{-1}. One strong band at around 1150 cm^{-1} in fingerprint region was found due to C-O-C stretching of polyethylene glycol. These are the common values found in all PEGylated cloxacillin, cephalexin and ciprofloxacin FTIR spectra due to common PEG 4000 presence in all.

H^1-NMR spectra of cloxacillin conjugated PEG 4000 showed signals at δ 1.25, 3.64 and 7.25-7.27 ppm. These signals are due to methyl protons of 6-aminopenicillenic acid of cloxacillin, (-O-CH_2-CH_2)- protons of PEG 4000 and phenyl ring protons of cloxacillin respectively. This proton NMR spectrum further confirms the synthesis of PEGylated cloxacillin conjugate.

H^1-NMR spectrum of cephalexin conjugated PEG 4000 showed signals at δ 1.26, 3.60-3.73 and 7.28-7.33 ppm. These are due to methyl protons of 7-aminocephalosporinic acid of cephalexin, (-O-CH_2-CH_2) - protons of PEG 4000 and phenyl ring protons of cephalexin respectively. This proton NMR spectrum further confirmed the synthesis of PEGylated cephalexin conjugate.

H^1-NMR spectrum of ciprofloxacin conjugated PEG 4000 showed signals at δ 1.25-1.36, 3.64 and 7.27 ppm. These are due to methylene protons of ciprofloxacin, (-O-CH_2-CH_2) - protons of PEG 4000 and phenyl ring protons of ciprofloxacin respectively. This proton NMR spectrum further confirmed the synthesis of PEGylated ciprofloxacin conjugate.

Thus in the light of these evidences it can be concluded that the PEGylated cloxacillin, cephalexin and ciprofloxacin were formed satisfactorily.

Drug-conjugated PEG-dendrimer complexes were synthesized easily by the use of para nitrophenylchloroformate activated PEGylated drugs. The reaction scheme of syntheses of drug derivatives is depicted in Scheme 2.

The synthesized drug derivatives were characterized by observing their physicochemical characteristics including spectral characters along with elemental analysis of nitrogen. The observations obtained were on predicted line. These drug derivatives showed different physical characters as compared to reactants. The nitrogen content found and calculated was almost similar as shown in Table 3.2. Spectroscopic data are recorded with interpretation in Tables 3.12-3.23.

The FTIR spectrums of drug-conjugated PEG-dendrimer shows almost similar bands as the most of the part of the compounds are same.

The main change found in the spectrum of drug-conjugated PEG and drug-conjugated PEG-dendrimer was the secondary amine band at around 3328 cm^{-1}, which confirms the bonding with dendrimer having lots of secondary amino groups. The primary amino group doublet bands in FTIR of dendrimer disappeared after forming drug-conjugated PEG-dendrimer, again confirming that the reaction took place in between primary amine of dendrimer and PEGylated drugs. These spectral changes were found in all the derivatized drugs (cloxacillin, cephalexin and ciprofloxacin).

H^1-NMR of cloxacillin-conjugated PEG-dendrimer showed four types of signals at δ 1.25-1.35, 2.17-2.18, 3.64-3.78 and 7.25-7.27 ppm. The signals at 1.25-1.35 confirmed the presence of methyl groups of cloxacillin which is absent in H^1-NMR of dendrimer alone. The peak at 2.17-2.18 ppm is due to protons of dendrimer which is absent in H^1-NMR spectrum of PEGylated cloxacillin, thus confirms the addition of dendrimer to PEGylated cloxacillin. The signals at 3.64-3.78 ppm are due to protons of PEG 4000 – ($O-CH_2-CH_2$)-, which are absent in H^1-NMR of dendrimer, confirming the conjugation of dendrimer with PEGylated cloxacillin. The signal at 7.25-7.27 ppm is due to protons of phenyl ring of cloxacillin, which is also present in H^1-NMR of PEGylated cloxacillin, further confirming PEGylated cloxacillin-dendrimer conjugation.

H^1-NMR of cephalexin-conjugated PEG-dendrimer shows four types of signals at δ 1.26-1.29, 1.63, 3.49-3.65 and 7.27-7.34 ppm. The signals at 1.26-1.29 confirms the presence of methyl group of cephalexin which is absent in H^1-NMR of dendrimer alone. The signal at 1.63 ppm is due to protons of dendrimer which is absent in H^1-NMR spectrum of PEGylated cephalexin, which confirms the addition of dendrimer to PEGylated cephalexin. The signals at 3.49-3.65 ppm are due to protons of PEG 4000 – ($O-CH_2-CH_2$)-, which are absent in H^1-NMR of dendrimer, confirming the conjugation of dendrimer with PEGylated cephalexin. The signals at 7.27-7.34 ppm is due to protons of phenyl ring of cephalexin, which is also present in H^1-NMR of PEGylated cephalexin, further confirming PEGylated cephalexin-dendrimer conjugation.

H^1-NMR of ciprofloxacin-conjugated PEG-dendrimer shows four types of signals at δ 1.25-1.36, 1.67, 3.49-3.65 and 7.27-7.37 ppm. The signal at 1.25-1.36 confirms the presence of methylene group of ciprofloxacin which is absent in H^1-NMR of dendrimer alone. The signal at 1.67 ppm is due to protons of dendrimer which is absent in H^1-NMR spectrum of PEGylated ciprofloxacin, thus confirms the addition of dendrimer to PEGylated ciprofloxacin. The signal at 3.49-3.65 ppm are due to protons of PEG 4000 – ($O-CH_2-CH_2$)-, which are absent in H^1-NMR of dendrimer, confirming the conjugation of dendrimer with PEGylated ciprofloxacin. The signal at 7.27-7.37 ppm is due to protons of phenyl ring of ciprofloxacin, which is also present in H^1-NMR of PEGylated ciprofloxacin, further confirming PEGylated ciprofloxacin-dendrimer conjugation.

Thus on the basis of results obtained in the characterization of drug derivatives, it can be concluded that the synthesized derivatives are in confirmation of the structures and the reactions went on to the predictions.

REFERENCE:

1. Egon Buhleier, Winfried Wehner, Fritz Vögtle (1978). ""Cascade"- and "Nonskid-Chain-like" Syntheses of Molecular Cavity Topologies". Synthesis (2): 155–158 (1978)
2. U.S. Patent 4,289,872.
3. U.S. Patent 4,410,688.
4. U.S. Patent 4,507,466.
5. D. A. Tomalia, H. Baker, J. Dewald, M. Hall, G. Kallos, S. Martin, J. Roeck, J. Ryder and P. Smith "A New Class of Polymers: Starburst-Dendritic Macromolecules". Polymer Journal 17: 117(1985).
6. "Treelike molecules branch out - chemist Donald A. Tomalia synthesized first dendrimer molecule - Chemistry - Brief Article". Science News. 1996.
7. George R. Newkome, Zhongqi Yao, Gregory R. Baker, Vinod K. Gupta (1985). "Micelles. Part 1. Cascade molecules: a new approach to micelles. A [27]-arborol". J. Org. Chem. 50 (11): (2003).
8. Hawker, C. J.; Fréchet, J. M. J. "Preparation of polymers with controlled molecular architecture. A new convergent approach to dendritic macromolecules". J. Am. Chem. Soc. 112 (21): 7638, (1990).
9. Zalipsky, S.; Gilon, C.; Zilkha, A. Attachment of drugs to polyethylene glycols Eur. Polym. J. 19, 1177-1183 (1983).
10. Silverstein RM; Webester FX, Spectrometric Identification of Organic Compounds, sixth edition published by John Wiley & Sons, Inc. 71-216, 1996.

Like life the researches too are endless, every step gives rise to another step to be completed. After successful syntheses and characterization of the new compounds the next step is to see whether these derivatives serve the purpose for what they had been synthesized. The purpose here was the enhancement of half-life of the drugs having short half-life. In search of the success many hypotheses are to be tried. Thus, the fate of the newly generated derivatives is to be seen in the in-vitro as well as in-vivo environment.

In order to provide the requisite, the chapter and studies are designed as following:

- *In vitro* activity of modified antibiotics (derivatized cloxacillin, cephalexin and ciprofloxacin) to prove their activity for the inhibition of bacterial growth.

- *In-vivo* assessment of half-life enhancement of derivatized drugs compared to drug alone.

4.1 IN-VITRO ACTIVITY

4.1.1 Introduction (Antimicrobial Evaluation)

The microbiological assay of an antibiotic is based upon a comparison of the inhibition of growth of micro-organisms by measured concentrations of the antibiotics under examination with that produced by known concentrations of a standard preparation of the antibiotic having a known activity. Two general methods are usually employed, the cylinder-plate (or cup-plate) method and the turbidimetric (or tube assay) method.

The cylinder-plate method (Method A) depends upon diffusion of the antibiotic from a vertical cylinder through a solidified agar layer in a Petri dish or plate to an extent such that growth of the added microorganism is prevented entirely in a zone around the cylinder containing a solution of the antibiotic. The turbidimetric method (Method B) depends upon the inhibition of growth of a microbial culture in a uniform solution of the antibiotic in a fluid medium that is favorable to its rapid growth in the absence of the antibiotic[1].

A. Cylinder-plate or Cup-plate method

Inoculate a previously liquefied medium appropriate to the assay with the requisite quantity of suspension of the micro organism, add the suspension to the medium at a temperature between 40° and 50° and immediately pour the inoculated medium into the petri dishes or large rectangular plates to give a depth of 3 to 4 mm (1 to 2mm for nystatin).

Ensure that the layers of medium are uniform in thickness, by placing the dishes or plates on a level surface. Store the prepared dishes or plates in a manner so as to ensure that no significant growth or death of the test organism occurs before the dishes or plates are used and that the surface of the agar layer is dry at the time of use.

Using the appropriate buffer solutions, prepare solutions of known concentrations of the standard preparation and solutions of the corresponding assumed of concentrations the antibiotic to be examined. Where directions have been given in the individual monograph for preparing the solutions, these should be followed and further dilutions made with buffer solution. Apply the solutions to the surface of the solid medium in sterile cylinders or in cavities prepared in the agar. The volume of solution added to each cylinder or cavity must be uniform and sufficient almost to fill the holes when these are used. When paper discs are used these should be sterilized by exposure of both sides under a sterilizing lamp and then impregnated with the standard solutions or the test solutions and placed on the surface of the medium. When Petri dishes are used, arrange the solutions of the Standard Preparation and the antibiotic under examination on each dish so that, they alternate around the dish and so that the highest concentrations of standard and test preparations are not adjacent. When plates are used, place the solutions in a Latin square design, if the plate is a square, or if it is not, in a randomized block design. The same random design should not be used repeatedly.

Leave the dishes or plates standing for 1 to 4 hours at room temperature or at 4°, as appropriate, as a period of preincubation diffusion to minimize the effects of variation in time between the application of the different solutions. Incubate them for about 18 hours at specified temperature. Accurately measure the diameters or areas of the circular inhibition zones and calculate the results. Selection of the assay design should be based on the requirements stated in the individual monograph.

B. Turbidimetric or Tube assay method

The method has the advantage of a shorter incubation period for the growth of the test organism (usually 3 to 4 hours) but the presence of solvent residues or other inhibitory substances affects this assay more than the cylinder plates assay and care should be taken to ensure freedom from such substances in the final test solutions. This method is not recommended for cloudy or turbid preparations.

Prepare five different concentrations of the standard solution for preparing the standard curve by diluting the stock solution of the Standard Preparation of the antibiotic and increasing stepwise in the ratio 4:5. Select the median concentration and dilute the solution of the substance being examined (unknown) to obtain approximately this concentration. Place 1 ml of each concentration of the standard solution and of the sample solution in each of the tubes in duplicate. To each tube add 9 ml of nutrient medium previously seeded with the appropriate test organism.

At the same time prepare three control tubes, one containing the inoculated culture medium (culture control), and another identical with it but treated immediately with 0.5 ml of *dilute formaldehyde solution* (blank) and a third containing uninoculated culture medium.

Place all the tubes, randomly distributed or in a randomized block arrangement, in an incubator or water-bath and maintain them at the specified temperature for 3 to 4 hours.

After incubation add 0.5 ml of *dilute formaldehyde solution* to each tube. Measure the growth of the test organism by determining the absorbance at about 530 nm of each of the solutions in the tubes against the blank.

In the present study, cup-plate method was used to compare the antibacterial activity of derivatized antibiotics to antibiotics alone to prove their efficacy in prohibition of bacterial growth.

Antimicrobial spectrum of selected drugs

Antimicrobial spectrum of cloxacillin:

Cloxacillin is penicillinase-resistant penicillin having a more narrow spectrum of activity than the natural penicillins. Their antimicrobial efficacy is aimed directly against penicillinase-producing strains of gram positive cocci, particularly *Staphylococcal* species like Staphylococcus aureus, Streptococcus pneumoniae, Streptococcus milleri. They are sometimes called anti-staphylococcal penicillins. There are documented strains of Staphylococcus that are resistant to these drugs (so-called methicillin-resistant *Staph*). While this class of penicillin do have activity against some other gram positive and gram negative aerobes and anaerobes, other antibiotics (penicillins and otherwise) are usually better choices. The penicillinase-resistant penicillins are inactive against *Rickettsia*, mycobacteria, fungi, *Mycoplasma* and viruses.

Antimicrobial spectrum of cephalexin:

Cefalexin is a beta-lactam antibacterial. It is bactericidal and acts similarly to benzylpenicillin by inhibiting synthesis of the bacterial cell wall. It is most active against Gram-positive cocci, and has moderate activity against some Gram-negative bacilli.

Sensitive Gram-positive cocci include both penicillinase-and non-penicillinase-producing staphylococci, although meticillin-resistant staphylococci are resistant; most streptococci are also sensitive, but not penicillin-resistant *Streptococcus pneumoniae;* enterococci are usually resistant. Some Gram-positive anaerobes are also susceptible. Cefalexin is usually inactive against *Listeria monocytogenes*.

Among Gram-negative bacteria cefalexin has activity against some Enterobacteriaceae including strains of *Escherichia coli*, *Klebsiella pneumoniae*, *Proteus mirabilis*, *Salmonella*, and *Shigella* spp., but not against *Enterobacter*, indole-positive *Proteus*, or *Serratia* spp. It is also active against *Moraxella catarrhalis* (*Branhamella catarrhalis*) and *Neisseria* spp., though *Haemophilus influenzae* is moderately resistant. *Bacteroides fragilis* and *Pseudomonas aeruginosa* are not sensitive and neither are mycobacteria, mycoplasma, and fungi.

Antimicrobial spectrum of ciprofloxacin:

Among Gram-positive aerobic bacteria, ciprofloxacin is active against staphylococci, including penicillinase-producing and penicillinase-nonproducing strains, and against some meticillin-resistant strains. Streptococci, in particular *Streptococcus pneumoniae* and enterococci, are less susceptible. Other Gram-positive bacteria sensitive to ciprofloxacin *in vitro* are *Bacillus anthracis* and *Corynebacterium* spp.

Among Gram-negative aerobic bacteria, ciprofloxacin is active *in vitro* against Enterobacteriaceae, including *Escherichia coli* and *Citrobacter*, *Enterobacter*, *Klebsiella*, *Proteus*, *Providencia*, *Salmonella*, *Serratia*, *Shigella*, and *Yersinia* spp. It is also active against *Pseudomonas aeruginosa*, but less so against other *Pseudomonas* spp. *Haemophilus ducreyi*, *H. influenzae*, *Moraxella catarrhalis* (*Branhamella catarrhalis*), and *Neisseria gonorrhoeae* are all very sensitive, including beta-lactamase-producing strains; *N. meningitidis* is also susceptible. Other Gram-negative aerobic bacteria reported to be sensitive to ciprofloxacin have included *Acinetobacter* spp., *Campylobacter* spp., *Gardnerella vaginalis*, *Helicobacter pylori*, *Legionella* spp., *Pasteurella multocida*, and *Vibrio* spp. Variable activity has been reported against *Brucella melitensis*.

Most anaerobic bacteria, including *Bacteroides fragilis* and *Clostridium difficile*, are resistant to ciprofloxacin, although some other *Clostridium* spp. may be susceptible.

Ciprofloxacin has some activity against mycobacteria, mycoplasmas, rickettsias, and the protozoan *Plasmodium falciparum*. *Chlamydia trachomatis* is moderately susceptible, and *Nocardia asteroides* and *Ureaplasma urealyticum* are usually considered to be resistant. The spirochaete *Treponema pallidum* and fungi are also resistant.

On the basis of antimicrobial spectrum of all the selected drugs it is found that all are showing good activity against penicillinase-producing strains of gram positive cocci, particularly *Staphylococcal* species such as Staphylococcus aureus. So we selected *Staphylococcus aureus* for screening of the derivatized drugs for their activity.

4.1.2 *Staphylococcus aureus*[2]

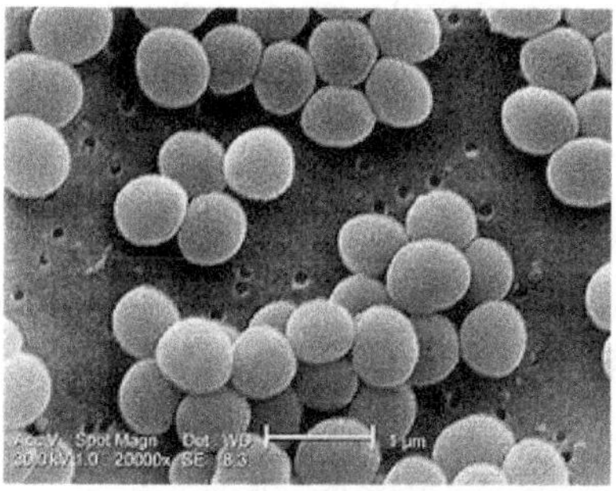

Figure 4.1 Scanning electron micrograph of *S. aureus*, 20,000 times enlargement, false color added

Scientific classification

Domain: Bacteria

Kingdom: Eubacteria

Phylum: Firmicutes

Class: Bacilli

Order: Bacillales

Family: Staphylococcaceae

Genus: Staphylococcus

Species: ***aureus***

Staphylococcus aureus meaning the "golden grape-cluster berry," and also known as "golden staph" and Oro staphira, is a facultative anaerobic Gram-positive coccal bacterium. It is frequently part of the skin flora found in the nose and on skin, and in this manner about 20% of the human populations are long-term carriers of *S. aureus*. S. aureus is the most common species of staphylococci to cause *Staph* infections. One of the reasons for this is a carotenoid pigment staphyloxanthin that is responsible for the characteristic golden colour of *S. aureus* colonies. This pigment acts as a virulence factor, with an antioxidant action that helps the microbe evade death by reactive oxygen species used by the host immune system.

S. aureus can cause a range of illnesses from minor skin infections, such as pimples, impetigo, boils (furuncles), cellulitis folliculitis, carbuncles, scalded skin syndrome, and abscesses, to life-threatening diseases such as pneumonia, meningitis, osteomyelitis, endocarditis, toxic shock syndrome (TSS), chest pain, bacteremia, and sepsis. Its incidence is from skin, soft tissue, respiratory, bone, joint, endovascular to wound infections. It is still one of the five most common causes of nosocomial infections, often causing post surgical wound infections. Each year, some 500,000 patients in American hospitals contract a staphylococcal infection.

Methicillin-resistant *S. aureus*, abbreviated MRSA and often pronounced "*mer*-sa", is one of a number of greatly-feared strains of *S. aureus* which have become resistant to most antibiotics. MRSA strains are most often found associated with institutions such as hospitals, but are becoming increasingly prevalent in community-acquired infections. A recent study by the Translational Genomics Research Institute showed that nearly half (47%) of the meat and poultry in U.S. grocery stores were contaminated with *S. aureus*, with more than half (52%) of those bacteria resistant to antibiotics.

4.1.3 Media

4.1.3.1 Mueller Hinton Agar[3-10] (MHA)

A solid medium originally designed for the isolation of pathogenic Neisseria species, now widely used for antibiotic susceptibility testing (including sulfonamides).

Composition:

Ingredients	**Grams/Litre**
Beef infusion solids	4.0
Starch	1.5
Casein hydrolysate	17.5
Agar	15.0

Final pH 7.4 +/- 0.2 at 37°C

Store prepared media below 8°C, protected from direct light. Store dehydrated powder, in a dry place, in tightly-sealed containers at 2-25°C.

Directions:

Suspend 38 g in 1 litre of distilled water, bring to the boil to dissolve the medium completely and sterilize by autoclaving at 121°C for 15 minutes.

Principle and Interpretation:

Mueller Hinton Agar is recommended for the disk diffusion method of antibiotic susceptibility testing. Mueller Hinton medium is recommended by FDA, World Health Organization and National Committee for Clin. Lab. Standards (NCCLS) for testing most commonly encountered aerobic and facultative anaerobic bacteria in food and clinical material. The medium shows good batch-to-batch reproducibility. It is low in sulfonamide, trimethoprim, and tetracycline inhibitors and yields satisfactory growth of most non-fastidious pathogens.

Beef infusion and Casein provide nitrogenous compounds, vitamins, carbon, sulphur and amino acids in Mueller Hinton media. Starch is added to absorb any toxic metabolites produced.

Paper discs impregnated with certain amount of specific antibiotics are placed on the surface of the medium. The plates are incubated and the zones of inhibition around each disc are measured. Different factors influence the disc diffusion susceptibility tests as inoculum concentration, agar depth, disc potency, medium pH and beta-lactamase production by test organisms.

For testing streptococci, supplementation with 5% defibrinated sheep or horse blood is recommended. Mueller Hinton media should be supplemented with 2% NaCl for testing methicillin or oxacillin against staphylococci. Mueller Hinton media with Rabbit Serum is used for the susceptibility of microorganisms to sulfonamides and trimethoprim. Antagonism to sulfonamide activity is demonstrated by para-aminobenzoic acid (PABA) and its analogs. Reduced activity of trimethoprim is demonstrated on medium possessing high levels of thymidine. The PABA and thymine/thymidine content of Mueller Hinton media is reduced to a minimum.

Cultural characteristics after 24 hours at 35°C.

Organisms (ATCC)	**Growth**
Escherichia coli (25922)	+++
Staphylococcus aureus (25923)	+++
Pseudomonas aeruginosa (27853)	+++
Neisseria meningitidis (13090)	+++
Streptococcus faecalis (29212)	+++

4.1.3.2 Mueller Hinton Broth[3-10] (MHB)

A liquid medium for antibiotic susceptibility studies [Minimum Inhibitory Concentration (MIC)-determination].

Composition:

Ingredients	Grams/Litre
Beef infusion solids	4.0
Starch	1.5
Casein hydrolysate	17.5

Final pH 7.4 +/- 0.2 at 37°C

Store prepared media below 8°C, protected from direct light. Store dehydrated powder, in a dry place, in tightly-sealed containers at 2-25°C.

Directions:

Dissolve 23 g in 1 litre of distilled water. Sterilize by autoclaving at 121°C for 15 minutes.

Principle and Interpretation:

Mueller Hinton Broth is used for determining minimal inhibitory concentrations. Mueller Hinton medium is recommended by FDA, World Health Organization and NCCLS for testing most commonly encountered aerobic and facultative anaerobic bacteria in food and clinical material. The medium shows good batch-to-batch reproducibility, it is low in sulfonamide, trimethoprim, and tetracycline inhibitors and yields satisfactory growth of most non-fastidious pathogens.

Beef infusion and Casein provide nitrogenous compounds, vitamins, carbon, sulphur and amino acids in Mueller Hinton media. Starch is added to absorb any toxic metabolites produced.

For testing streptococci, supplementation with 5% defibrinated sheep or horse blood is recommended. Mueller Hinton media should be supplemented with 2% NaCl for testing methicillin or oxacillin against staphylococci. Mueller Hinton media with Rabbit Serum is used for the susceptibility of microorganisms to sulfonamides and trimethoprim. Antagonism to sulfonamide activity is demonstrated by para-aminobenzoic acid (PABA) and its analogs. Reduced activity of trimethoprim is demonstrated on medium possessing high levels of thymidine. The PABA and thymine/thymidine content of Mueller Hinton media is reduced to a minimum.

Cultural characteristics after 24 hours at 35°C.

Organisms (ATCC)	**Growth**
Escherichia coli (25922)	+++
Staphylococcus aureus (25923)	+++
Pseudomonas aeruginosa (27853)	+++
Neisseria meningitidis (13090)	+++
Streptococcus faecalis (29212)	+++

4.1.4 Experimental

Stock culture of *Staphylococcus aureus* (ATCC 33862) was maintained at 4°C on slants of nutrient agar. Active cultures for the study was prepared by transferring a loopful of cells from the stock culture to test tube of Mueller-Hinton broth (MHB) and this tube was incubated without agitation for 24 h at 37°C. After getting growth, the cultures were diluted with fresh MHB to an inoculum size of 10^6 colony forming units/ml[11].

The disc diffusion method was used to know the antibacterial activity of the drugs[12]. In-vitro antibacterial activity was determined by using Mueller-Hinton Agar (MHA) medium. The MHA plates were prepared by pouring 15ml of sterile molten medium into sterile Petri dishes. The plates were allowed to solidify and a lawn of bacterial culture was made on MHA plates (Using an asceptic technique, a sterile swab was placed into the broth culture of staphylococcus aureus and then gently removed excess liquid by gently pressing the swab against the inside of the tube. By using this swab, Mueller-Hinton agar plate was streaked. To obtain uniform growth, the plate was streaked with the swab in one direction and then rotated at 90° and streaked the plate again in that direction. The rotation was repeated 3 times. Then the plate was allowed to dry for approximately 5 minutes).

Identical concentrations of antibiotics [5 mcg/disc cloxacillin, 30 mcg/disc cephalexin and 5 mcg/disc ciprofloxacin] and derivatized antibiotics [equivalent to 5 mcg/disc cloxacillin, 30 mcg/disc cephalexin and 5 mcg/disc ciprofloxacin] were loaded on 6 mm sterile filter paper discs. (Whatman No.1 filter papers were obtained and disks of about 6 mm were cut out from the filter papers. These were wrapped in foil paper and sterilized in the oven at 160°C for 1 h).

In addition, some sterile filter paper discs were soaked in sterile distilled water. Those discs were placed on the surface of the dried inoculated MHA plates, by using flame-sterilized forceps; each disc was gently pressed to the agar to ensure that the disc is attached to the agar and the drug was allowed to diffuse for 2 h at room temperature during which time diffusion of the antibiotic into the medium occurred[13]. Then the plates were kept for incubation at 37°C for 24 h. At the end of incubation period, inhibition zones formed around the discs were measured with the help of zone reader in mm.

For each antibiotic, three MHA plates were used in a similar fashion. The results were represented as average zone of inhibition for each antibiotic used in this study. The antibacterial activity was evaluated by measuring inhibition zones of bacterial growth. In the study, discs soaked in distilled water served as negative control and standard antibiotic discs was used as positive control.

4.1.5 Antimicrobial activity observations

Table 4.1 Comparative antibacterial study of cloxacillin and derivatized cloxacillin

Name of micro-organism	Zone of Inhibition (mm)		
	Std. Clox.[a]	Der. Clox.[b]	D.W.[c]
Staphylococcus aureus	22	20	0

a- Standard Cloxacillin, b- Derivatized Cloxacillin, c- Distilled Water

Table 4.2 Comparative antibacterial study of cephalexin and derivatized cephalexin

Name of micro-organism	Zone of Inhibition (mm)		
	Std. Ceph.[a]	Der. Ceph.[b]	D.W.[c]
Staphylococcus aureus	17	16	0

a- Standard Cephalexin, b- Derivatized Cephalexin, c- Distilled Water

Table 4.3 Comparative antibacterial study of ciprofloxacin and derivatized ciprofloxacin

Name of micro-organism	Zone of Inhibition (mm)		
	Std. Cipro.[a]	Der. Cipro.[b]	D.W.[c]
Staphylococcus aureus	30	29	0

a- Standard Ciprofloxacin, b- Derivatized Ciprofloxacin, c- Distilled Water

4.2 In-Vivo Activity

4.2.1 Introduction

In vivo (Latin for "within the living") is experimentation using a whole, living organism as opposed to a partial or dead organism, or an in vitro ("within the glass", i.e., in a test tube or petri dish) controlled environment. Animal testing and clinical trials are two forms of in vivo research. In vivo testing is often employed over in vitro because it is better suited for observing the overall effects of an experiment on a living subject. This is often described by the maxim in vivo veritas.[14]

In vivo testing is also known as animal experimentation, animal research, and Animal testing, is the use of non-human animals in experiments. Worldwide it is estimated that the number of vertebrate animals—from zebrafish to non-human primates—ranges from the tens of millions to more than 100 million used annually.[15] Invertebrates, mice, rats, birds, fish, frogs, and animals not yet weaned are not included in the figures; one estimate of mice and rats used in the United States alone in 2001 was 80 million.[16] Most animals are euthanized after being used in an experiment.[17] Sources of laboratory animals vary between countries and species; most animals are purpose-bred, while others are caught in the wild or supplied by dealers who obtain them from auctions and pounds.[18]

4.2.2 Animals

Wistar albino rats (Weight 200-300g) of either sex were employed in present study. They were fed on standard laboratory chow (Kishan Feeds Ltd., New Delhi, India) and had free access to tap water *ad libitum*. All experimental protocols were followed according to Animal Ethical Committee in Gyan Vihar School of Pharmacy, with Protocol No. 16.

4.2.2 In-vivo studies of derivatized cloxacillin

Twelve male Albino Wistar rats (200-300g) were randomly assigned to two treatment groups for i.v. dosing (six per group). The rats were lightly anaesthetized with ether prior to the insertion of a silastic catheter into the jugular vein, which was then exteriorized to the back of the neck. The same catheter was used for drug administration and for blood sampling. All rats were alert at the time of dosing. Each rat in group A received a 30 mg/kg i.v. bolus dose of cloxacillin in water. Blood samples (0.2 ml) were taken just prior to dosing and at 05, 15, 30, 60, 90, 120, 180, 240, 300, 400, 500, 600, 800, 1000, 1200, 1400 and 1600 min. following drug administration. Each rat in group B received Derivatized cloxacillin i.v. bolus dose equivalent to 30 mg/kg of cloxacillin. Blood samples were obtained at the same time as those outlined for group A. Blood was collected in heparinized polypropylene tubes and immediately centrifuged at 2000 rpm for 15 minutes. The plasma was harvested and stored at - 20°C pending analysis. Plasma concentrations of cloxacillin and derivatized cloxacillin were quantified by a sensitive and validated high-performance liquid chromatographic procedure[19]. Young Lin Autochro-3000 HPLC system was used with stainless steel column 4.6×250 mm, packed with octadecylsilyl silica gel 5μm. Composition of mobile phase was a mixture of 74 volumes of 100 mM potassium hydrogen phosphate solution and 26 volumes of acetonitrile. Flow rate was 1ml/minute. UV-Visible detector was set at 220 nm and a 20 μl loop injector was used. The lower limit of quantification was 0.12 μg/mL of plasma.

The cloxacillin and derivatized cloxacillin were extracted from their plasma samples by mixing the samples with precipitating agent (1% formic acid in acetonitrile) in a ratio of 1:3 v/v. The precipitated proteins were then removed by centrifugation at 3000 rpm for 10 minutes, and upper organic layer was transferred to a clean tube and dried under nitrogen flow at room temperature. The residue was reconstituted with 100 μL of mobile phase and 20 μL of aliquot was injected into chromatograph.

Standard curve for cloxacillin determination in plasma samples:

Plasma calibrators (0.2 µg/mL to 10 µg/mL) for calibration curve were prepared in drug free control plasma. Ten concentrations (excluding blank value) defined the calibration curve. The linearity of the calibration curve was verified from 0.2 µg/mL to 10 µg/mL for cloxacillin in plasma. The correlation coefficient was found more than 0.999. The limit of quantitation was found 120 ng/mL for plasma. The relation between response and concentration was demonstrated to be continuous and reproducible. This calibration curve was used to calculate the concentrations of unknown samples assayed at different time intervals. The calibration curve covered the entire range of expected concentrations.

Table 4.4 Cloxacillin Concentration in drug free control plasma Vs Mean Area

S.No.	Cloxacillin concentrations in drug free control plasma (ng/mL)	Mean Area (mV*Sec)
1.	200	16.23
2.	400	31.62
3.	800	62.28
4.	1200	93.12
5.	1600	121.52
6.	2000	154.22
7.	4000	306.82
8.	6000	460.12
9.	8000	609.38
10.	10000	763.60

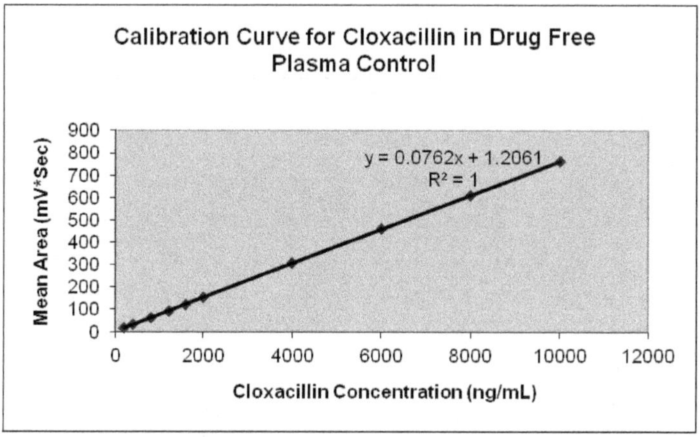

Fig 4.2 Calibration curve of cloxacillin in drug free control plasma

To check whether the drug dendrimer complex (DDC) interfere in the analysis or not; chromatograms of plasma blank, plasma with drug, plasma with DDC and plasma with DDC & drug were taken. The chromatograms obtained are shown in Figure 4.3 to 4.7 for cloxacillin.

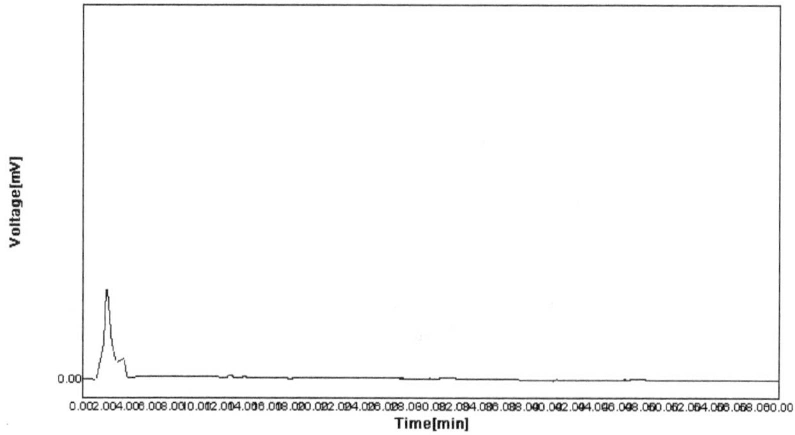

Fig 4.3 Plasma Blank for cloxacillin

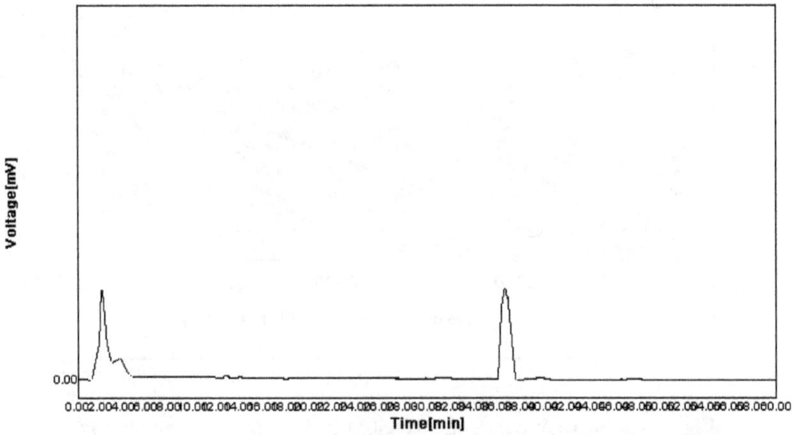

Fig 4.4 Plasma with cloxacillin

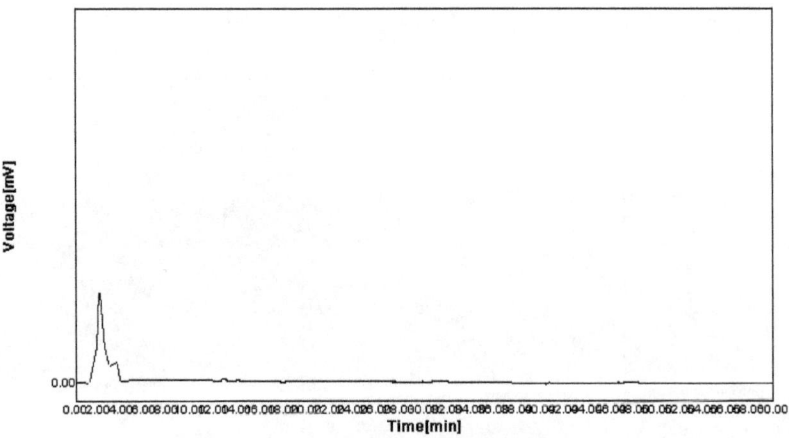

Fig. 4.5 Plasma with DDC

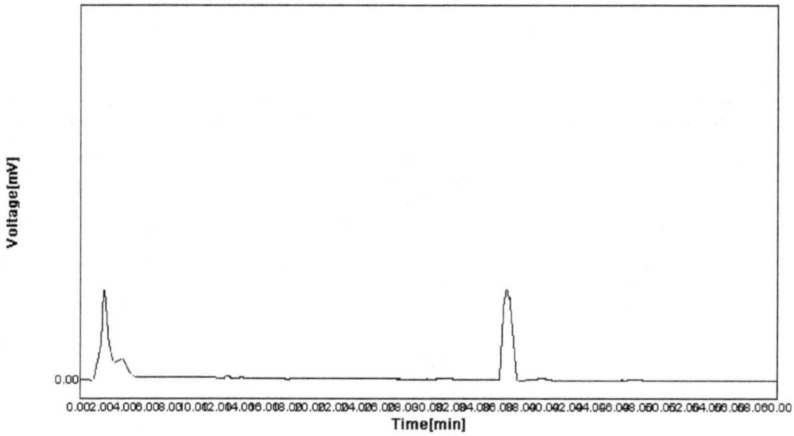

Fig. 4.6 Plasma with DDC & Cloxacillin

Table 4.5 Concentrations of cloxacillin and cloxacillin released from DDC obtained by HPLC analysis of plasma samples collected at different time intervals

S.No.	Time (Minutes)	Cloxacillin Concentration (ng/ml)	Derivatized Cloxacillin Concentration (ng/ml)
1.	05	7000	-
2.	15	3550	130
3.	30	1760	160
4.	60	470	280
5.	90	125	440
6.	120	-	560
7.	180	-	800
8.	240	-	990
9.	300	-	1160
10.	400	-	1380
11.	500	-	1480
12.	600	-	1520
13.	800	-	1510
14.	1000	-	1260
15.	1200	-	760
16.	1400	-	150
17.	1600	-	-

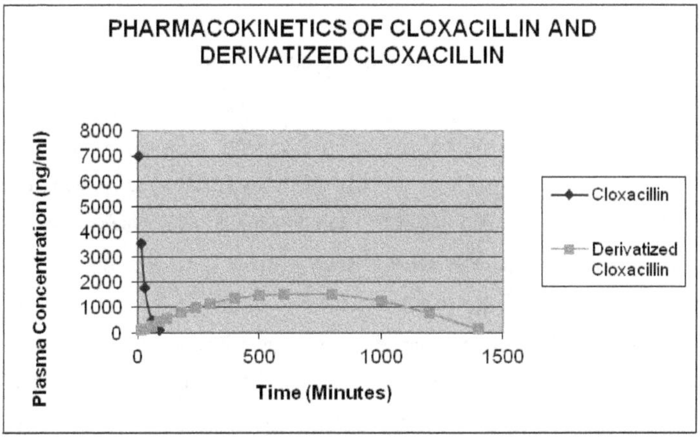

Fig. 4.7 Mean plasma concentrations of cloxacillin and derivatized cloxacillin following intravenous administration

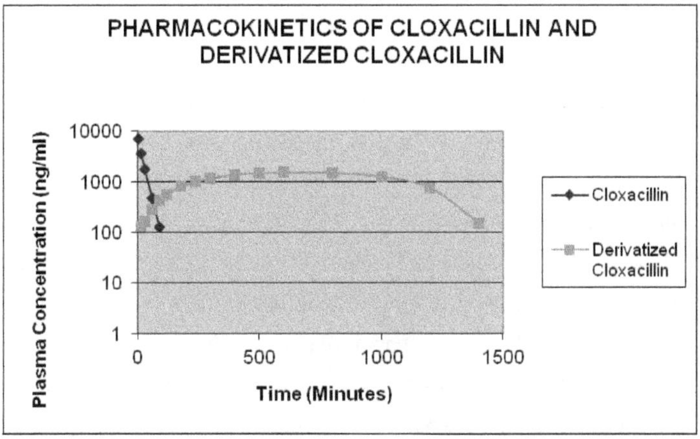

Fig. 4.8 Mean plasma concentrations of cloxacillin and derivatized cloxacillin following intravenous administration (log scale)

4.2.3 In-vivo studies of derivatized cephalexin

Twelve male Albino Wistar rats (200-300g) were randomly assigned to two treatment groups for i.v. dosing (six per group). The rats were lightly anaesthetized with ether prior to the insertion of a silastic catheter into the jugular vein, which was then exteriorized to the back of the neck. The same catheter was used for drug administration and for blood sampling. All rats were alert at the time of dosing. Each rat in group A received a 20 mg/kg i.v. bolus dose of cephalexin in water. Blood samples (0.2 ml) were taken just prior to dosing and at 05, 15, 30, 60, 90, 120, 180, 240, 300, 400, 500, 600, 800, 1000, 1200, 1400 and 1600 min. following drug administration. Each rat in group B received Derivatized cephalexin i.v. bolus dose equivalent to 20 mg/kg of cephalexin. Blood samples were obtained at the same time as those outlined for group A. Blood was collected in heparinized polypropylene tubes and immediately centrifuged at 2000 rpm for 15 minutes. The plasma was harvested and stored at - 20°C pending analysis. Plasma concentrations of cephalexin and derivatized cephalexin were quantified by a sensitive and validated high-performance liquid chromatographic procedure[20]. Young Lin Autochro-3000 HPLC system was used with a stainless steel column 4.6×250 mm, packed with octadecylsilyl silica gel 5µm (C-18 reversed-phase). Composition of mobile phase was a mixture of acetonitrile-methanol-acetate buffer of pH 4.2 (10: 10: 80 %). Flow rate was 1.4 mL/minute. UV-Visible detector was set at 254 nm and a 20 µl loop injector was used. The lower limit of quantification was 1 µg/mL of plasma.

The cephalexin and derivatized cephalexin were extracted from their plasma samples by mixing the samples with precipitating agent (1% zinc sulphate solution). The precipitated proteins were then removed by centrifugation at 3000 rpm for 10 minutes, and upper organic layer was transferred to a clean tube and dried under nitrogen flow at room temperature. The residue was reconstituted with 100 µL of mobile phase and 20 µL of aliquot was injected into chromatograph.

Standard curve for cephalexin determination in plasma samples:

Plasma calibrators (5 µg/mL to 50 µg/mL) for calibration curve were prepared in drug free control plasma. Six concentrations (excluding blank value) defined the calibration curve. The linearity of the calibration curve was verified from 5µg/mL to 50 µg/mL for cephalexin in plasma. The correlation coefficient was 0.9997. The limit of quantitation was 1 µg/mL for plasma. The relation between response and concentration was demonstrated to be continuous and reproducible. This calibration curve was used to calculate the concentrations of unknown samples assayed at different time intervals. The calibration curve covered the entire range of expected concentrations.

Table 4.6 Cephalexin concentrations in drug free control plasma Vs. Mean Area

S.No.	Cephalexin concentrations in drug free control plasma (µg/mL)	Mean Area (mV*Sec)
1.	05	25.68
2.	10	48.36
3.	20	99.72
4.	30	146.08
5.	40	196.44
6.	50	248.80

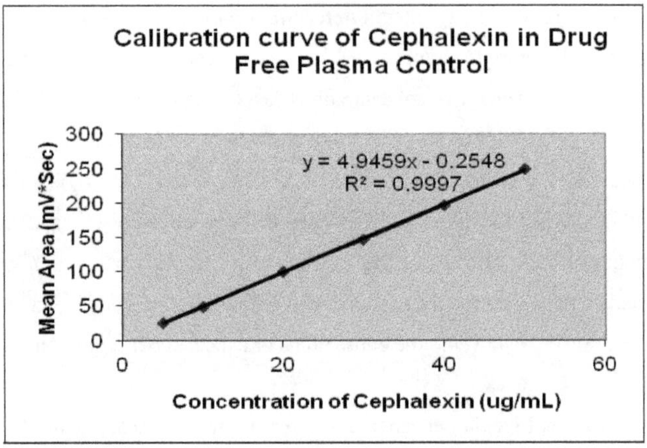

Fig. 4.9 Calibration curve of cephalexin in drug free control plasma

To check whether the drug dendrimer complex (DDC) interfere in the analysis or not chromatograms of plasma blank, plasma with drug, plasma with DDC and plasma with DDC & drug were taken. The chromatograms obtained are shown in Figure 4.10 to 4.13 for cephalexin.

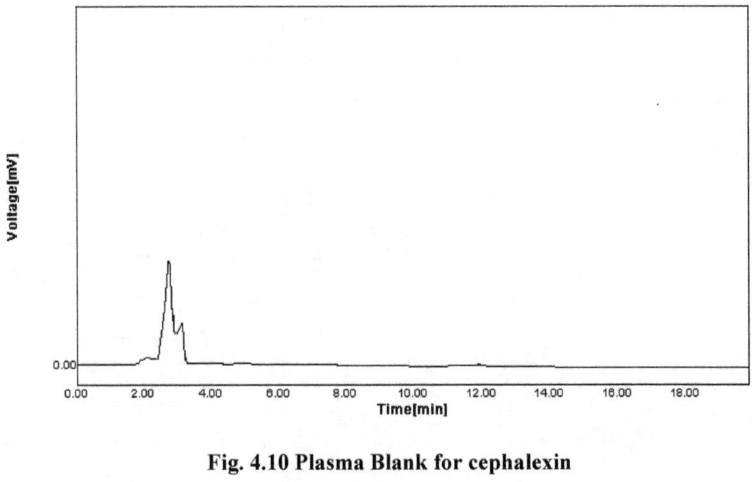

Fig. 4.10 Plasma Blank for cephalexin

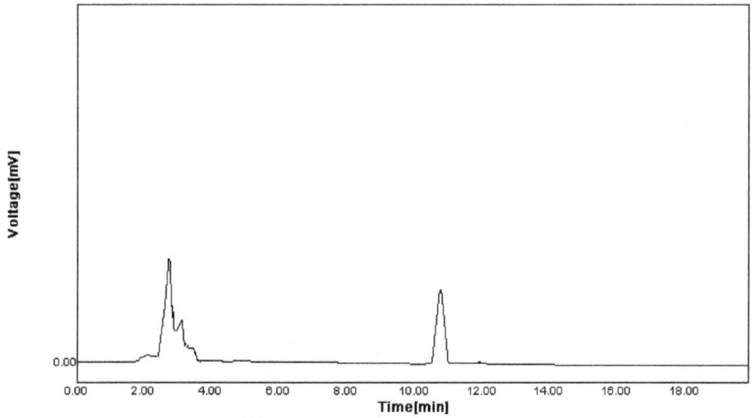

Fig. 4.11 Plasma with cephalexin

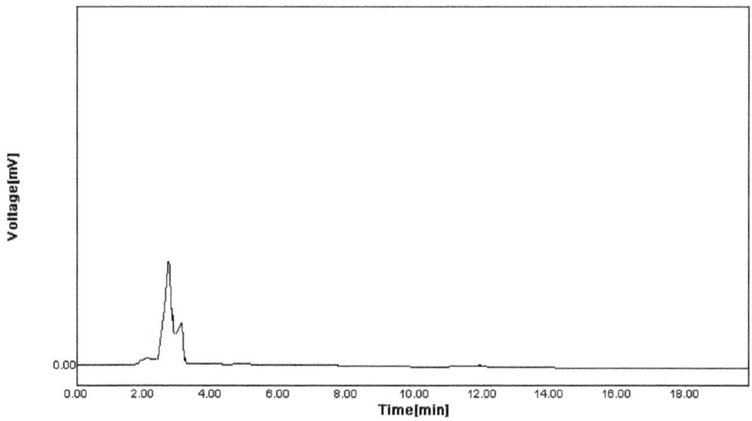

Fig 4.12 Plasma with DDC

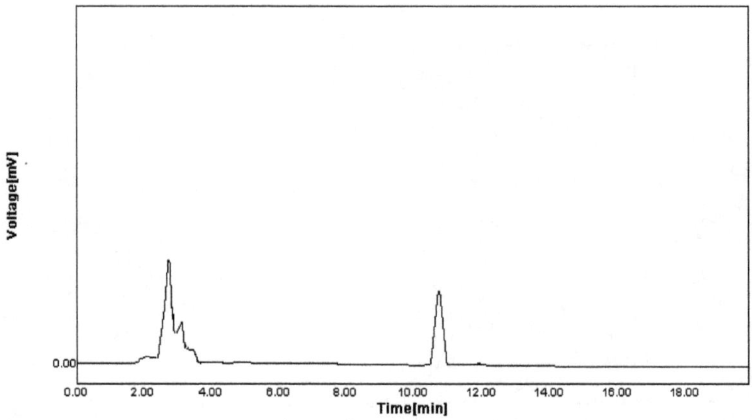

Fig. 4.13 Plasma with DDC & Cephalexin

Table 4.7 Concentrations of cephalexin and cephalexin released from DDC obtained by HPLC analysis of plasma samples collected at different time intervals

S.No.	Time (Minutes)	Cephalexin Concentration (μg/ml)	Derivatized Cephalexin Concentration (μg/ml)
1.	05	25	-
2.	15	12	-
3.	30	06	01
4.	60	1.5	02
5.	90	-	3.2
6.	120	-	4.2
7.	180	-	5.6
8.	240	-	6.5
9.	300	-	07
10.	400	-	7.6
11.	500	-	08
12.	600	-	7.9
13.	800	-	7.4
14.	1000	-	6.2
15.	1200	-	4.3
16.	1400	-	2.2
17.	1600	-	-

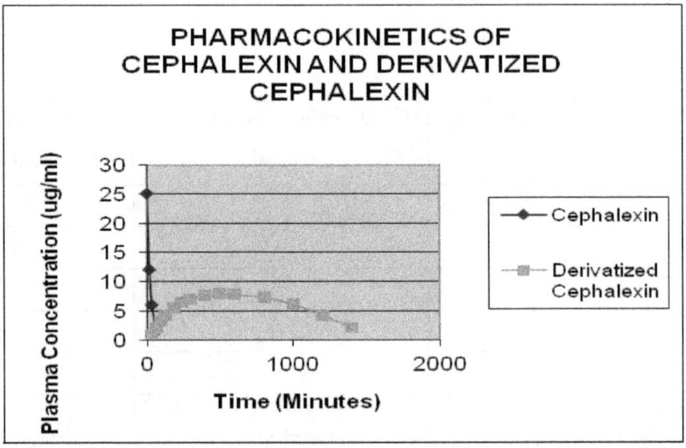

Fig 4.14 Mean plasma concentrations of cephalexin and derivatized cephalexin following intravenous administration

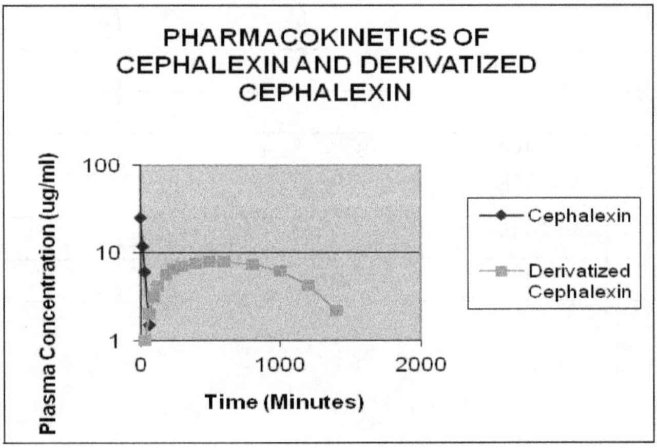

Fig 4.15 Mean plasma concentrations of cephalexin and derivatized cephalexin following intravenous administration (log scale)

4.2.3 In-vivo studies of derivatized ciprofloxacin

Twelve male Albino Wistar rats (200-300g) were randomly assigned to two treatment groups for i.v. dosing (six per group). The rats were lightly anaesthetized with ether prior to the insertion of a silastic catheter into the jugular vein, which was then exteriorized to the back of the neck. The same catheter was used for drug administration and for blood sampling. All rats were alert at the time of dosing. Each rat in group A received a 5 mg/kg i.v. bolus dose of ciprofloxacin in water. Blood samples (0.2 ml) were taken just prior to dosing and at 05, 15, 30, 60, 90, 120, 180, 240, 300, 400, 500, 600, 800, 1000, 1200, 1400, 1600 and 1800 min. following drug administration. Each rat in group B received Derivatized ciprofloxacin i.v. bolus dose equivalent to 5 mg/kg of ciprofloxacin. Blood samples were obtained at the same time as those outlined for group A. Blood was collected in heparinized polypropylene tubes and immediately centrifuged at 1000 rpm for 15 minutes. The plasma was harvested and stored at - 20°C pending analysis. Plasma concentrations of ciprofloxacin and derivatized ciprofloxacin were quantified by a sensitive and validated high-performance liquid chromatographic procedure[21]. Young Lin Autochro-3000 HPLC system was used with stainless steel column 4.6×250 mm, packed with octadecylsilyl silica gel 5µm (C-18 reversed-phase). Composition of mobile phase was a mixture of 0.01 M phosphate buffer (pH = 2.6, adjusted with concentrated orthophosphoric acid) and methanol in a ratio of 82 and 18 v/v respectively. Flow rate was 1.5 mL/minute. Uv-visible detector was set at 277 nm and a 20 µl loop injector was used. The lower limit of quantification was 20 ng/mL of plasma.

The ciprofloxacin and derivatized ciprofloxacin were extracted from their plasma samples by mixing the samples with precipitating agent (1% formic acid in acetonitrile) in a ratio of 1:3 v/v. The precipitated proteins were then removed by centrifugation at 3000 rpm for 10 minutes, and upper organic layer was transferred to a clean tube and dried under nitrogen flow at room temperature. The residue was reconstituted with 100 µL of mobile phase and 20 µL of aliquot was injected into chromatograph.

Standard curve for ciprofloxacin determination in plasma samples:

Plasma calibrators (0.05 μg/mL to 8 μg/mL) for calibration curve were prepared in drug free control plasma. Six concentrations (excluding blank value) defined the calibration curve. The linearity of the calibration curve was verified from 5μg/mL to 50 μg/mL for ccephalexin in plasma. The correlation coefficient was 0.9997. The limit of quantitation was 1 μg/mL for plasma. The relation between response and concentration was demonstrated to be continuous and reproducible. This calibration curve was used to calculate the concentrations of unknown samples assayed of different time intervals. The calibration curve covered the entire range of expected concentrations.

Table 4.8 Ciprofloxacin concentrations in drug free control plasma vs. Mean Area

S.No.	Ciprofloxacin concentrations in drug free control plasma (ng/mL)	Mean Area (mV*Sec)
1.	50	19.12
2.	100	29.34
3.	1000	286.39
4.	2000	572.02
5.	4000	1140.42
6.	8000	2272.12

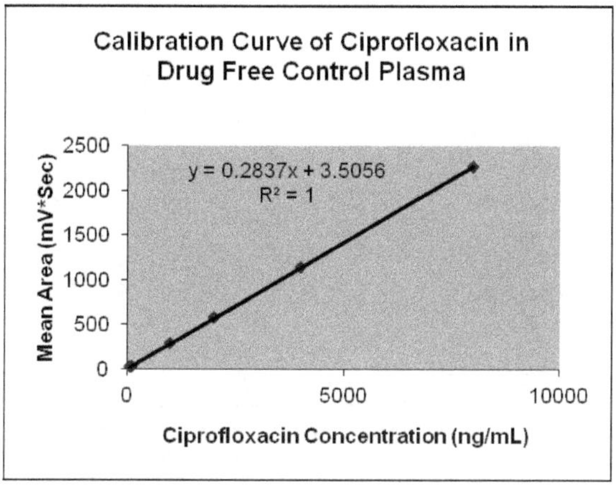

Fig. 4.16 Calibration curve of ciprofloxacin in drug free control plasma

To check whether the drug dendrimer complex (DDC) interferes in the analysis or not chromatograms of plasma blank, plasma with drug, plasma with DDC and plasma with DDC & drug were taken. The chromatograms obtained are shown in Figure 4.17 to 4.20 for ciprofloxacin.

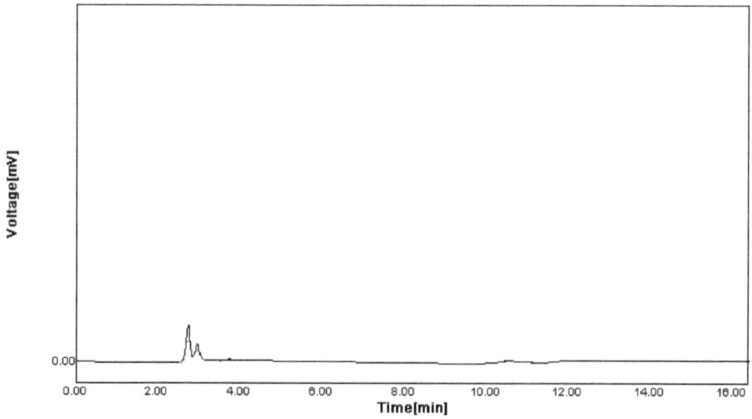

Fig 4.17 Plasma Blank for Ciprofloxacin

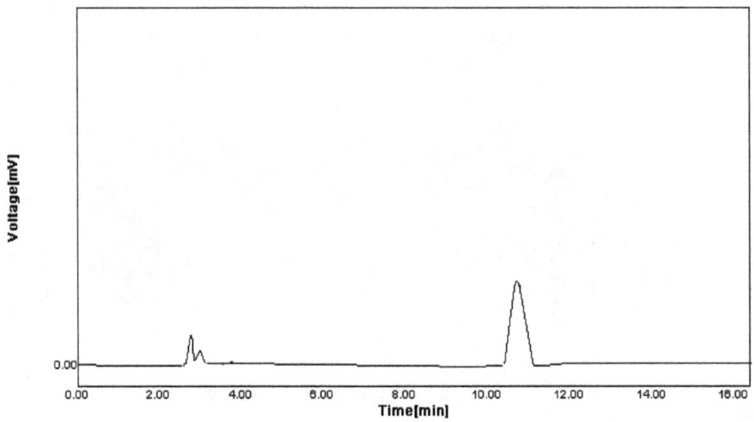

Fig. 4.18 Plasma with ciprofloxacin

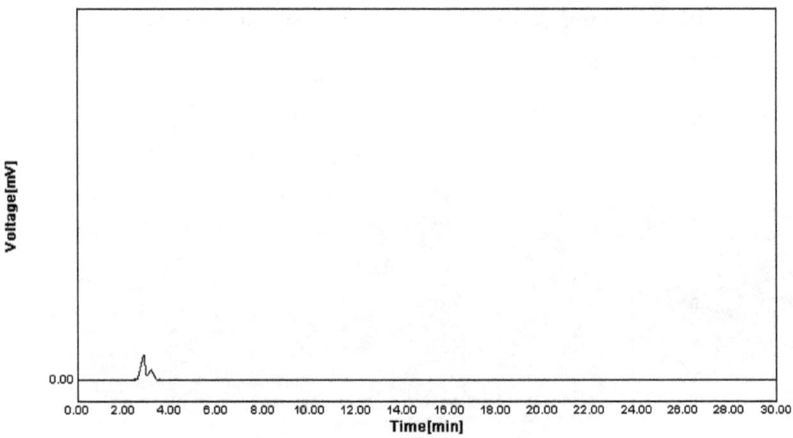

Fig. 4.19 Plasma with DDC

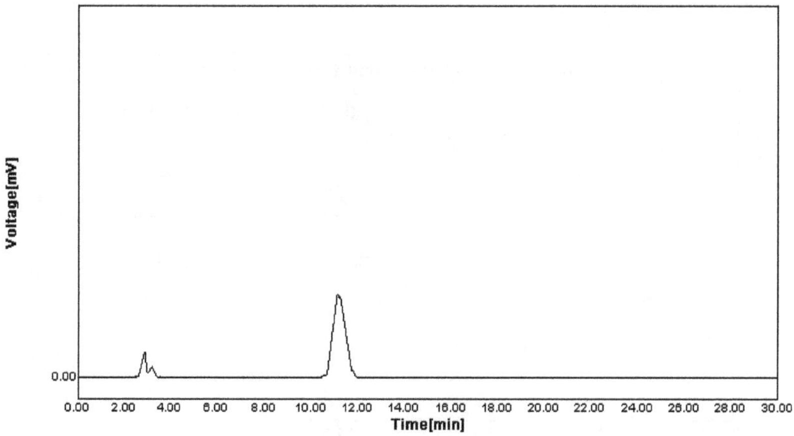

Fig. 4.20 Plasma with DDC & Ciprofloxacin

Table 4.9 Concentrations of ciprofloxacin and ciprofloxacin released from DDC obtained by HPLC analysis of plasma samples collected at different time intervals

S.No.	Time (Minutes)	Ciprofloxacin Concentration (ng/ml)	Derivatized Ciprofloxacin Concentration (ng/ml)
1.	05	4920	-
2.	15	3996	30
3.	30	3109	59
4.	60	2305	140
5.	90	1902	240
6.	120	1100	300
7.	180	580	480
8.	240	312	620
9.	300	140	720
10.	400	59	860
11.	500	-	950
12.	600	-	980
13.	800	-	1000
14.	1000	-	970
15.	1200	-	900
16.	1400	-	760
17.	1600	-	600
18.	1800	-	360
19.	2000	-	-

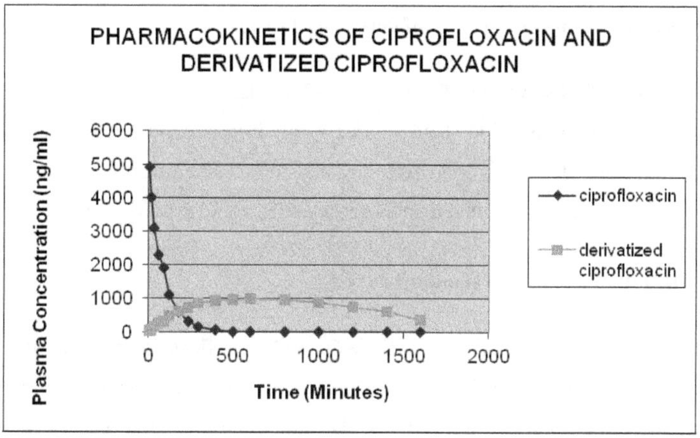

Fig 4.21 Mean plasma concentrations of ciprofloxacin and derivatized ciprofloxacin following intravenous administration

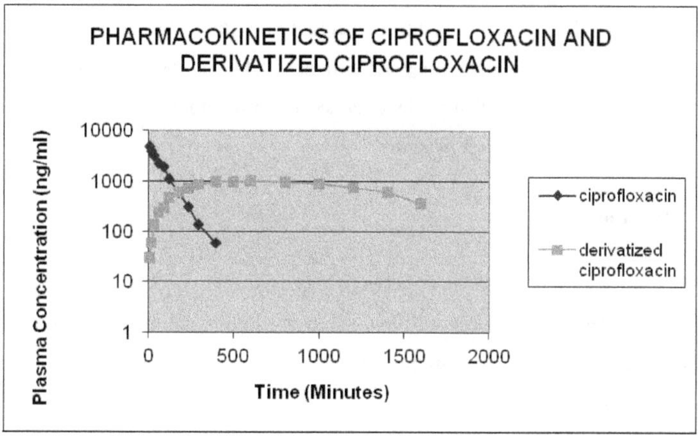

Fig. 4.22 Mean plasma concentrations of ciprofloxacin and derivatized ciprofloxacin following intravenous administration (log scale).

Result & Discussion

➢ Results of in-vitro activity of derivatized drugs

On the basis of observations (Table 4.1, 4.2 & 4.3) found in in-vitro activity of derivatized drugs compared to standard drug alone, it was found that zone of inhibition obtained by both category of drugs (standard and derivatized drugs) were almost similar. That means drug derivatization did not alter the antibacterial activity of drugs.

➢ Result of analysis of standard curve

Calibration curve for cloxacillin, cephalexin and ciprofloxacin in drug free control plasma were found linear between concentration and mean area. The correlation coefficient for all curves were 0.999. By the help of these calibration curves, concentrations of unknown samples assayed at different time intervals were calculated.

➢ Interference

On the basis of chromatograms (fig. 4.3 to 4.6 for cloxacillin, fig. 4.10 to 4.13 for cephalexin and 4.17 to 4.20 for ciprofloxacin) it was found that peak obtained due to plasma is not interfering with drug as well as DDC was not showing any peak in chromatograms that proved that peaks obtained in chromatograms were only due to the released drugs from DDC in rat plasma.

➢ Half-life

On the basis of graphs obtained in-between mean plasma concentration of drugs, drug released from derivatized drugs and time taken in elimination of them, half-life's were calculated, calculated results are summarized in Table 4.10.

Table 4.10 Half-life Enhancement Data from In-vivo Experiments

S.No.	Name of Drug	$t_{1/2}$ (Rat Plasma) Drug alone	$t_{1/2}$ (Rat Plasma) Derivatized Drug	Half-life Enhancement
1.	Cloxacillin	12 Minutes	600 Minutes	50 Folds
2.	Cephalexin	12.5 Minutes	730 Minutes	58.4 Folds
3.	Ciprofloxacin	15 Minutes	990 Minutes	66 Folds

Results showing dramatically increase in half-life of derivatized drugs compared to drug alone when administered intravenously into albino rats.

References

1. Microbiological Assay of Antibiotics, Indian Pharmacopoeia 2007, vol. 1, Government of India, Ministry of Health & Family Welfare, Published by the Indian Pharmacopoeia Commission, Ghaziabad, 2007, 45.

2. http://en.wikipedia.org/wiki/staphylococcus_aureus. (last visited on 5/7/2011)

3. NCCLS Approved Standard: ASM-2, Performance Standards for Antimicrobic disc SusceptibilityTests, 2nd ed., National Committee for Clin. Lab. Standards (1979)

4. NCCLS M7-T Tentative Standard, National Committee for Laboratory Standards (1983)

5. Bauer et al, Am. J. Clin. Path., 45, 493 (1966)

6. Ericsson and Sherris, Acta. Pathol. Microbiol., Scand. Sec. B. Suppl., 217, 1 (1971)

7. Present Status and Future Work, WHO Sponsored collaborative study, Chicago (1967)

8. J.H. Müller, J. Hinton, Proc. Soc. Exptl. Biol. 48, 330 (1941)

9. G.M. Eliopoulus, et al., Enhancement of cefotoxamine and other cephalosporins against Enterococcus faecalis by blood supplemented Mueller-Hinton agar, Diagn. Microbiol. Infect. Dis.12, 149 (1989);

10. R.D. Jenkins, et al., J. Clin. Microbiol. 22, 369 (1985).

11. Collins CH, Lynes PM, Grange JM. Microbiological methods. 7th edn, Butterwort-Hinemann Ltd, Britain, 1995, 175-190.

12. Bauer RW, Kirby MDK, Sherris JC, Turck M. Antibiotic susceptibility testing by standard single disc diffusion method. Am. J. Clin. Pathol., 45, 493-496(1966).

13. Bhaskar VH, Kumar M, Sangameswaran B, Balakrishnan BR. Antimicrobial activity of some 4- Thiazolidine derivatives. Pharmacist, 2, 1-5 (2007).

14. http://www.sciencemag.org/products/lst_20070622.dtl Life Science Technologies Cell Signaling: In Vivo Veritas--Science Magazine, 2007. (last visited on 5/7/2011)

15. Meredith Cohn, "Alternatives to Animal Testing Gaining Ground," The Baltimore Sun 26 August 2010.

16. Carbone, Larry. *What Animals Want*. Oxford University Press, 2004, p. 26.

17. Carbone, Larry. *What Animals Want*. Oxford University Press, 2004, p. 22.

18."Use of Laboratory Animals in Biomedical and Behavioral Research", Institute for Laboratory Animal Research, The National Academies Press, 1988.

19. Teare FW, Kwan RH, Spino M, Macleod SM. High-pressure liquid chromatographic assay of cloxacillin in serum and urine. J Pharm Sci., 71, 938-941 (1982).

20. Najib NW et al. High Performance liquid chromatographic analysis of cephalexin in serum and urine. Journal of Clinical Pharmacy and Therapeutics; 12, 419-426 (1987)

21. Amini M.; Khanavi M; Shafiee A; Simple High Performance Liquid Chromatographic Method for Determination of Ciprofloxacin in Human Plasma. Iranian Journal of Pharmaceutical Research 2, 99-101 (2004).

Therapeutically active agents, however, often suffer from number of shortcomings which limit and complicate their use. A particular problem is short half life of drugs. After administration to the patient, a drug may be so rapidly cleared from the body by metabolic or other pathways or otherwise biologically inactivated so that only a relatively small percentage of the drug administered actually has a therapeutic effect. For example many over the counter pain relievers like ibuprofen and medications that are used as tranquilizers like benzodiazepines have notoriously short half lives.

To compensate for this problem, it is common practice to increase the dose of the drug and/ or to prolong its period of administration and/ or to shorten the interval between doses so that the therapeutically effective concentration of the drug in the patient is maintained for a period sufficient to achieve the desired result.

These procedures are useful but have their own limitations. Increasing the dosage may be limited, for example, in the case of intramuscular administration, by the bolus which can be tolerated. Many drugs have toxic side effects which may limit the dosage duration or interval which can be safely used. In some cases, promising drugs cannot be used because side reactions are so severe that an effective therapeutic dose cannot be safely administered. The need to administer multiple small doses of a drug or to use continuous infusion techniques increases the cost of treatment and the burden on hospital personnel, and of course, adds to the patient's discomfort. Accordingly there exists a need for means by which the therapeutically active concentration of a drug after administration is maintained for a longer time.

Synthetic macromolecules are often employed as drug carriers to improve overall pharmacokinetic properties of drugs and to enhance their therapeutic effects. Recently dendrimers have attracted much attention in drug delivery because of their unique structures. Compared with linear polymers, dendrimers are well-defined globular highly branched macromolecules.

Summary & Conclusion

Their many accessible reactive end groups at the surface make it possible to tailor dendrimers' chemical and physical properties through proper chemical modification. Characteristics of dendritic structures, including toxicity, interactions with foreign objects (e.g., cells, opsonins), routes for cellular uptake, and intracellular fate will most likely be governed by the imparted surface groups. In contrast, such properties of conventional polymeric carriers may vary depending on their preferred folding pattern in a particular environment. Thus, a judicious choice of surface groups is crucial to optimize the pharmacological effects of a dendrimer-based drug delivery system.

We have designed and synthesized a drug-delivery scaffold based on new ethylene diamine tetra acetic acid (EDTA) core poly amidoamine (PAMAM) dendrimer having 16 primary amine groups on surface (Scheme1).

The incorporation of PEG chains into the dendritic structure was taken up because it can yield a number of biologically and pharmacokinetically desirable properties such as improved biocompatibility, reduced immunogenicity, prolonged half-life, increased water solubility, and enhanced structural stability, as reported in previous work.

We selected Cloxacillin, Cephalexin and Ciprofloxacin as model drugs having short half lives and a carboxylic acid group to attach to PEG-PAMAM star polymer. The linkage between these selected drugs and PEG is formed by ester bond (Scheme 2). Since it is believed that a carboxylic acid group is essential for the antibacterial activity of these drugs, hydrolysis release for drugs coupling with star polymer via ester bonds was studied. In case of PEG derivatives it was found that the renal clearance decreases with an increase in MW, with most dramatic change occurring near MW 30,000. Therefore, since a longer circulating lifetime of PEG-conjugated drugs can be achieved by increasing the MW of the polymeric agent that prevents rapid renal excretion. The star based drug-delivery systems could perform in a fashion to increase drug circulation time in the body and may provide more stability.

In the synthetic part first of all novel EDTA based PAMAM dendrimers were prepared using EDTA as a starting material.

The synthetic reactions performed were as following:

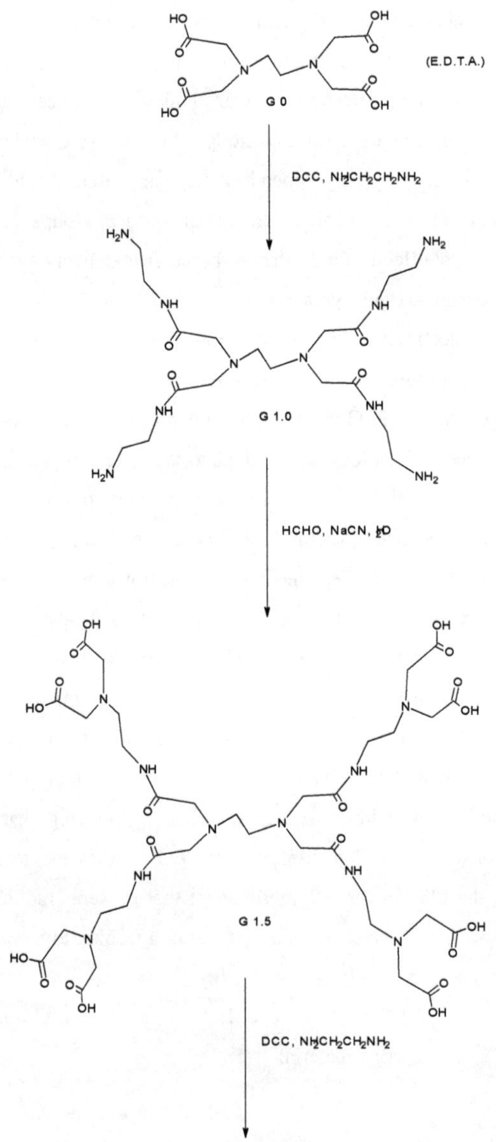

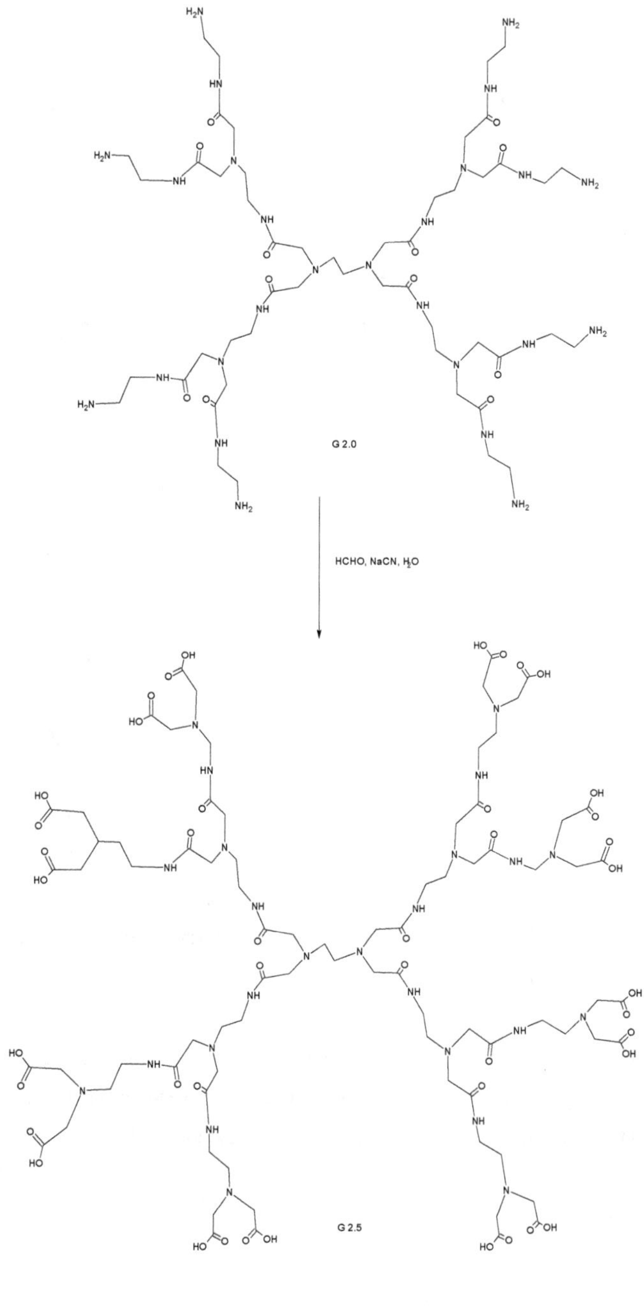
G 2.0
HCHO, NaCN, H_2O
G 2.5

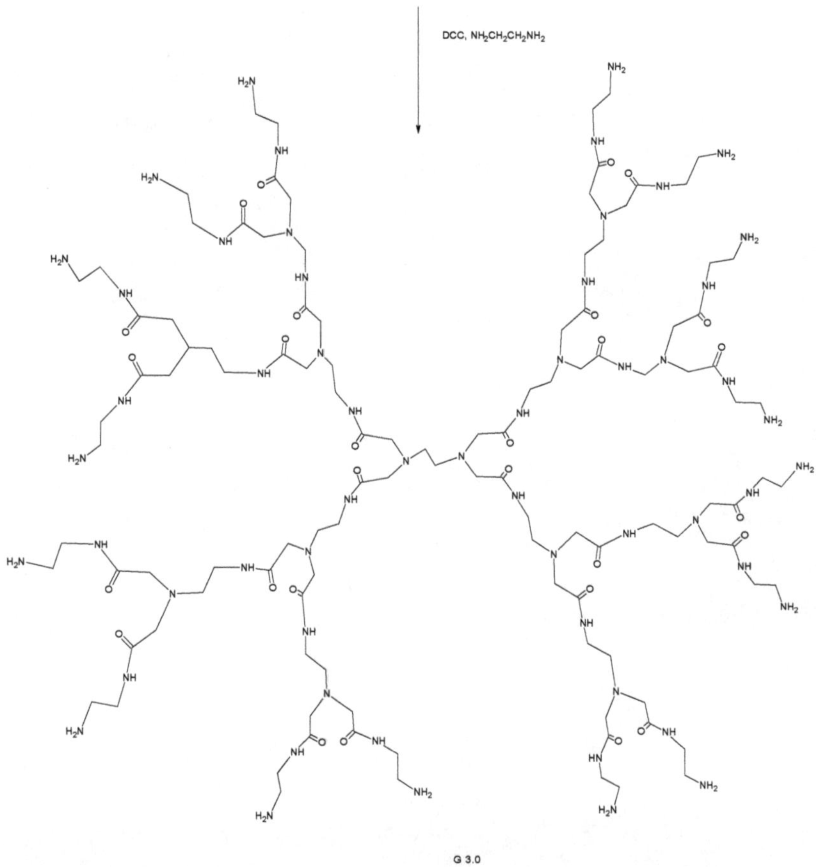

Synthetic Pathway of EDTA core PAMAM dendrimer (G 3.0) having 16 free primary amine groups

Selected drugs (cloxacillin, cephalexin, and ciprofloxacin) were conjugated with poly ethylene glycol 4000 via ester bond formation between carboxylic acid group of drugs and hydroxyl group of PEG 4000. The synthetic steps used were as following:

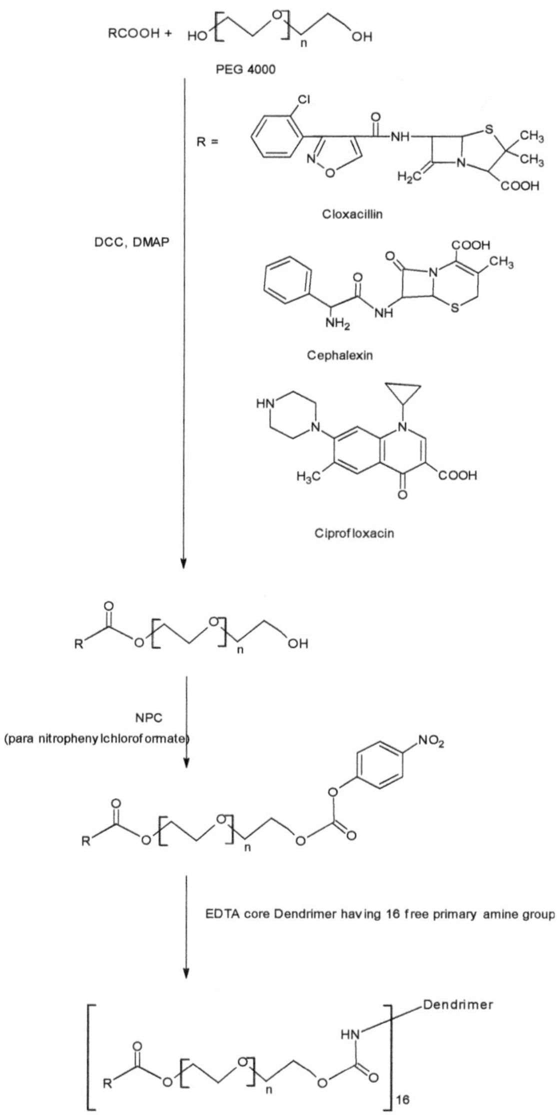

Synthetic steps used in preparation of drug-PEG 4000-dendrimer complex

Finally PAMAM dendrimer with EDTA core containing 16 primary amine surface groups connecting MW 4000 poly ethylene glycol and selected drugs were attached to the end of polyethylene glycol, were synthesized. Structures of final derivatized drugs are as following:

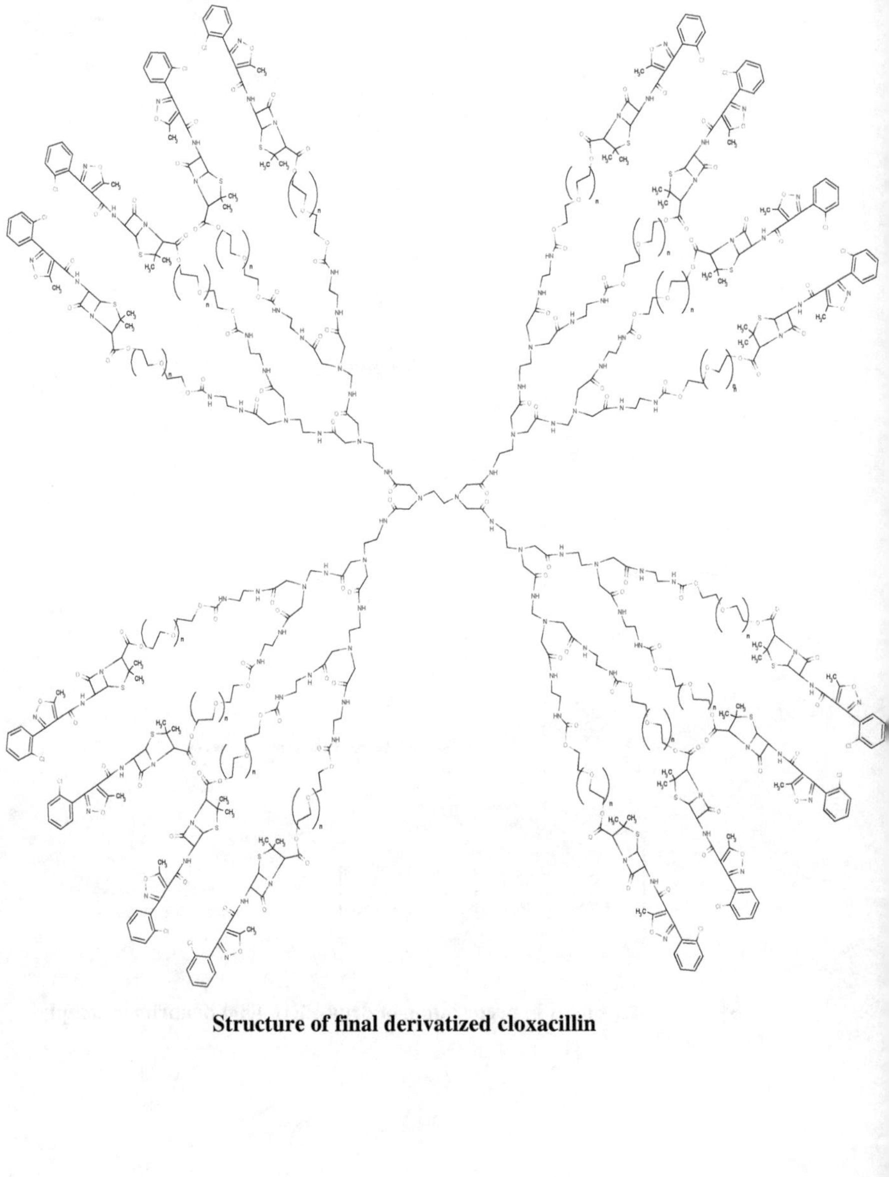

Structure of final derivatized cloxacillin

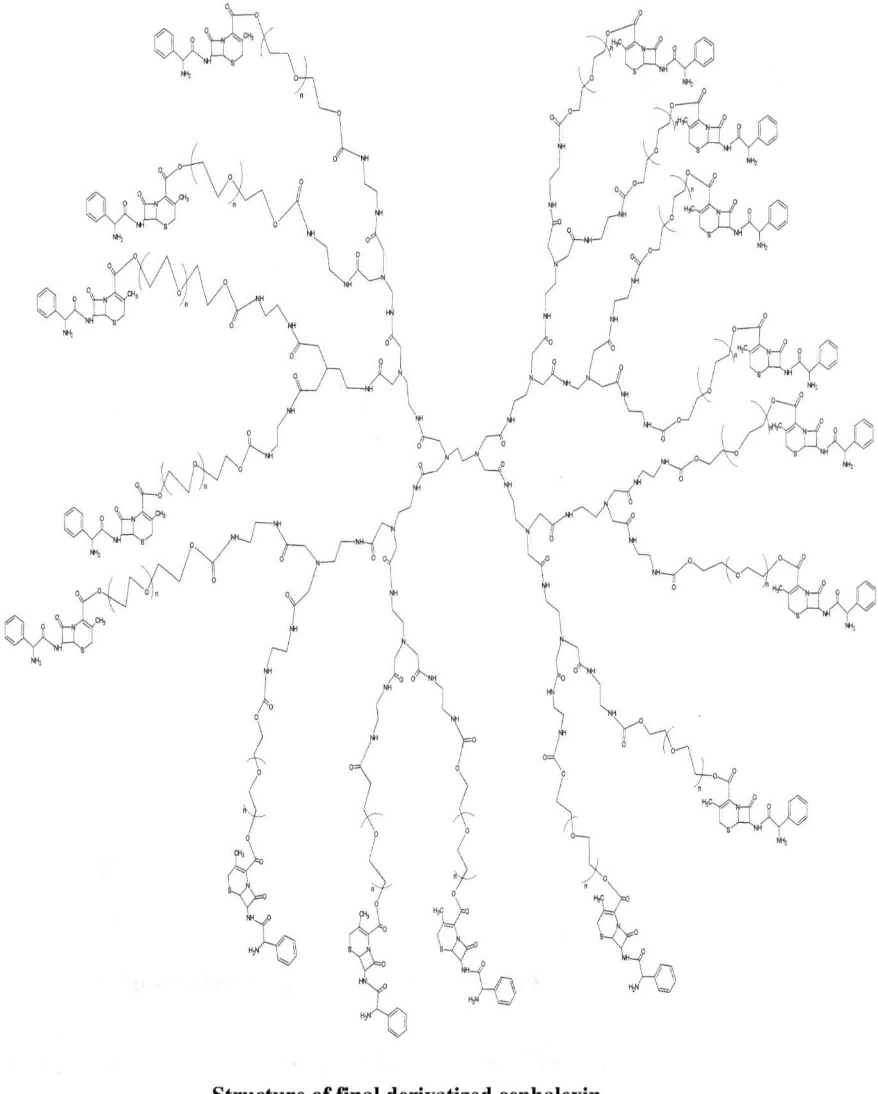

Structure of final derivatized cephalexin

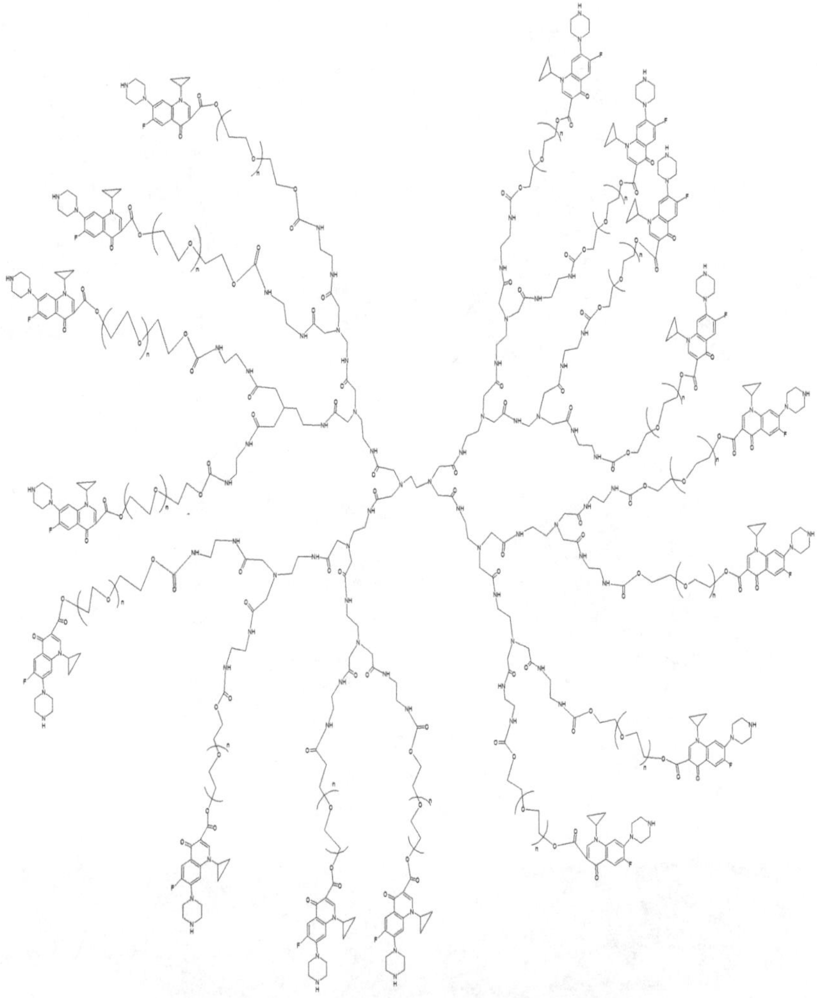

Structure of final derivatized ciprofloxacin

Characterization of the intermediates and drug-star polymer conjugates were done with the help of physicochemical and spectral characterization. Molecular weight enhancements of derivatized drugs were found as following:

Table: 5.1 Increase in molecular weight after drug derivatization

S.No.	Name of Drug	Mol.Wt. of Drug (Daltons)	Mol.Wt. of Derivatized Drug (Daltons)
1.	Cloxacillin	435.881	73,160
2.	Cephalexin	347.39	71,736
3.	Ciprofloxacin	331.34	71,480

After synthesis of derivatized drugs their In-vitro & In-vivo evaluations were performed. In order to prove the activity of modified antibiotics (derivatized cloxacillin, cephalexin and ciprofloxacin) for the inhibition of bacterial growth, their in vitro antibacterial activity were studied and compared with antibiotics alone using strain of *Staphylococcus aureus* by cup-plate method. In- vitro antibacterial activity was determined by using Mueller-Hinton Agar and Mueller-Hinton broth medium.

These derivatized drugs and standard disk of drugs (cloxacillin, cephalexin and ciprofloxacin) produced more or less similar zones of inhibition, which indicates that derivatized drugs retain antibacterial activity at its equivalent dose. Therefore the modification of drugs through esterification did not alter their antimicrobial activity. Comparative antibacterial study of drugs and derivatized drugs are shown in Table 4.1, 4.2 & 4.3.

In-vivo studies were performed by using male Wistar albino rats (Weight 200-300g). They were fed on standard laboratory chow and had free access to tap water *ad libitum.* Initially standard curve for each drug were made for the concentration determination of drug in plasma samples using selected method.

To investigate pharmacokinetic parameters, cloxacillin, cephalexin, ciprofloxacin and derivatized Cloxacillin, cephalexin, ciprofloxacin were intravenously injected into rats.

Plasma samples were collected at different time intervals and analyzed by validated HPLC methods. The modified antibiotics demonstrated dramatically greater half-life than antibiotics alone. Graphical representation of mean plasma concentrations of drugs alone and derivatized drugs following intravenous administration (log scale) are as following:

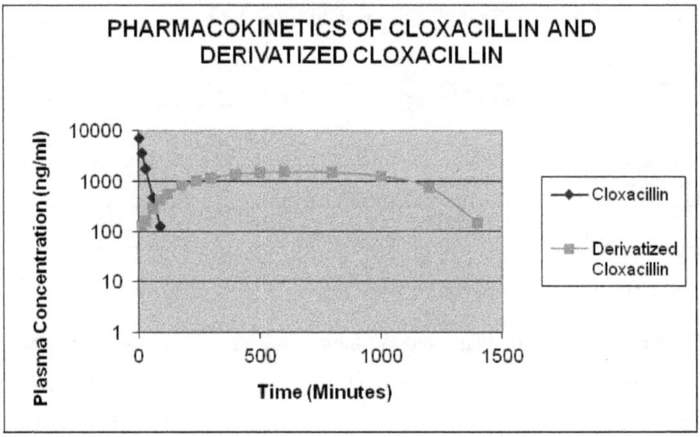
PHARMACOKINETICS OF CLOXACILLIN AND DERIVATIZED CLOXACILLIN
Plasma Concentration (ng/ml)
10000
1000
100
10
1
0
500
1000
1500
Time (Minutes)
Cloxacillin
Derivatized Cloxacillin

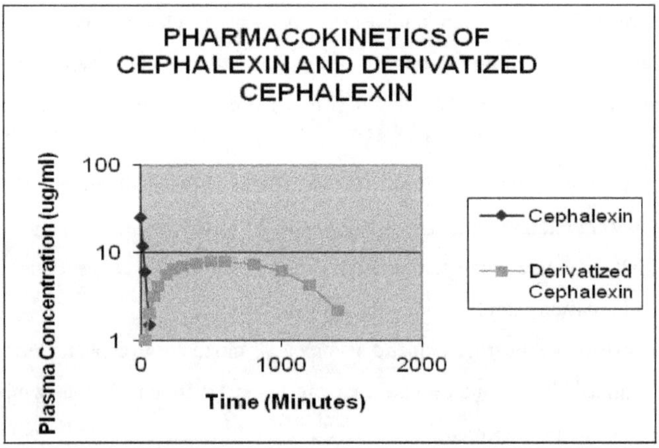
PHARMACOKINETICS OF CEPHALEXIN AND DERIVATIZED CEPHALEXIN
Plasma Concentration (ug/ml)
100
10
1
0
1000
2000
Time (Minutes)
Cephalexin
Derivatized Cephalexin

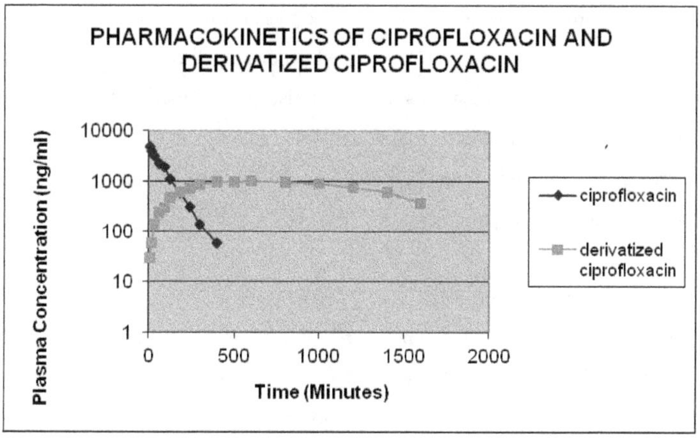

On the basis of graph obtained in-between mean plasma concentration of drugs & derivatized drugs and time taken in elimination of them half-life was calculated. Calculated results are as following:

Half-life Enhancement Data from In-vivo Experiments

S.No.	Name of Drug	$t_{1/2}$ (Rat Plasma) Drug alone	$t_{1/2}$ (Rat Plasma) Derivatized Drug	Half-life Enhancement
1.	Cloxacillin	12 Minutes	600 Minutes	50 Folds
2.	Cephalexin	12.5 Minutes	730 Minutes	58.4 Folds
3.	Ciprofloxacin	15 Minutes	990 Minutes	66 Folds

The result of present study indicates that plasma half-life of derivatized drugs increased dramatically. Conjugation of PEGylated dendrimer onto drugs enables them to avoid the normal renal clearance mechanisms and also protect them from enzymatic degradation thereby leads to increased plasma half-life. Such a prolonged retention of drugs should reduce the dosing frequency needed to remain above therapeutically effective concentrations of drug.

Achievement of objectives

The study revealed that the experimental drug showed enhancement of the half-life to 50-66 times. This will lead to the effective utilization of drug, minimization of dose and frequency of administration. It will also improve patient convenience, compliance and health care cost.

RECOMMENDATIONS

In present study, cloxacillin, cephalexin and ciprofloxacin were coupled with EDTA core PAMAM dendrimer through PEG spacer. The drug delivery scaffold based on PEG-polyamidoamine star polymer proved feasible. The star polymers provided accessible ends which were used to chemically couple desired small molecules. The method described here could be extended to prepare star polymers with different PEG arm lengths and to couple different functional groups (drugs) of interest.

These studies suggest the use of these new PEG based polymer supports as a valuable alternative for enhancing biological half-life of drugs.

This methodology can be extended to many other classes of drugs (having short half-life) to improve their half-life and reducing their dosing frequency.

Title: Drug Derivatization for Enhancement of Half-Life.

Name of Candidate: Vivek Gupta

Name of Supervisors: Dr. R.K. Agrawal & Dr. A.K. Shrivastava

PUBLICATIONS

S.No.	Title	Authors Name	Journal	Publisher	Website
1.	Ciprofloxacin Derivatization For Enhancement Of Its Half-Life	Vivek Gupta, Anil K. Shrivastava, Ram K. Agrawal	International Journal of Pharmaceutical Research and Development (IJPRD)	Online	www.ijprd.com
2.	Cloxacillin Derivatization for the Enhancement of Half-Life	Vivek Gupta, Anil K. Shrivastava, Ram K. Agrawal	International Journal of Research in Pharmaceutical and Biomedical Sciences (IJRPBS)	Online	www.ijrpbs.com
3.	Strategies to Manage Drug Metabolism : A Review	Vivek Gupta, Anil K. Shrivastava, Ram K. Agrawal	International Journal of Research in Pharmaceutical and Biomedical Sciences (IJRPBS)	Online	www.ijrpbs.com

CPSIA information can be obtained
at www.ICGtesting.com
Printed in the USA
LVHW021429011222
734355LV00016B/899

9 781805 450719